MAKING SENSE OF VASCULAR ULTRASOUND

MAKING SENSE OF VASCULAR ULTRASOUND

A HANDS-ON GUIDE

Kenneth A Myers
MS FRACS FACS DDU(Vasc)
Consultant Vascular Surgeon, Epworth Hospital and Monash
Medical Centre; Consultant in Vascular Imaging,
Melbourne Vascular Ultrasound, Melbourne, Victoria, Australia

Amy Clough
BSc DMU(Vasc)
Senior Vascular Ultrasonographer, Melbourne Vascular
Ultrasound, Epworth Hospital, Melbourne, Victoria, Australia

A member of the Hodder Headline Group
LONDON

First published in Great Britain in 2004 by
Arnold, a member of the Hodder Headline Group,
338 Euston Road, London NW1 3BH

http://www.arnoldpublishers.com

Distributed in the United States of America by
Oxford University Press Inc.,
198 Madison Avenue, New York, NY 10016
Oxford is a registered trademark of Oxford University Press

British Library Cataloguing in Publication Data
A catalogue record for this book is available from the British Library

Library of Congress Cataloging-in-Publication Data
A catalog record for this book is available from the Library of Congress

ISBN   0 340 81009 2

1 2 3 4 5 6 7 8 9 10

Commissioning Editor: Joanna Koster
Development Editor: Sarah Burrows
Project Editor: Naomi Wilkinson
Production Controller: Lindsay Smith
Cover Design: Sarah Rees

Typeset in 10.5/13 RotisSerif by Charon Tec Pvt. Ltd, Chennai, India
Printed and bound in Italy

What do you think about this book? Or any other Arnold title?
Please send your comments to feedback.arnold@hodder.co.uk

CONTENTS

PREFACE

There has been an explosion of new technology for vascular ultrasound throughout the past 30 years. Basic black and white instruments of the mid-1980s have now been replaced by extremely sophisticated units that allow colour display of flow in two or three dimensions. These use both B-mode and Doppler assessment assisted by power and harmonic Doppler imaging with the promise of many new techniques to come. There is hardly a radiological, vascular surgical or vascular medical practice anywhere in the world that does not employ ultrasound scanning to evaluate their patients with arterial or venous disease. General ultrasound practitioners are having to learn the peculiar requirements of vascular ultrasound, its potentials and its limitations. Increasingly, ultrasound is also being used to guide the actual treatment of both arterial and venous disease. The entire balance between diagnosis by conventional arteriography, ultrasound and other imaging modalities is being re-evaluated to obtain the best value from each and allow them to complement each other. The major benefit of ultrasound is that it is non-invasive and relatively inexpensive. However, vascular ultrasound is complex and this can become overwhelming to those who are learning the art, and indeed to established practitioners. The aim of this book is to attempt to get to the heart of how to apply physical and physiological principles to obtain the best results for assessment at various sites. It is designed to be a practical hands-on book for rapid reference in the course of day-to-day practice. However, it is also anticipated that it will be a concise reference book for trainee sonographers learning the techniques and attempting to pass examinations. It is hoped that it will simplify the complex issues so as to make better sense of vascular ultrasound.

ACKNOWLEDGEMENTS

We gratefully acknowledge the assistance provided in producing this book from Cheryl Bass, Andrew Dickenson, Valerie Gregory, Joe Kiss, Greg Lammers, Maurice Molan, Jason Paige, Rhonda Rose, Ian Schroen, Debby Smith, Allen Tabor and Stephen Wood. We particularly acknowledge the advice and support from our colleagues Jane Browne, Jayne Chambers and Penny Koh. We are grateful for the helpful and highly professional support received from Sarah Burrows, Penny Howes and Joanna Koster at the Hodder Headline Group.

Colour artwork sponsored by Philips Ultrasound.

Postscript

We appreciate critical comments regarding improvements, corrections and additions for future editions. Please contact us to make any suggestions that you see fit at: Kenneth Myers, Suite 5.1, 32 Erin Street, Richmond, Melbourne, Victoria, 3121, Australia.

LIST OF ABBREVIATIONS

AAA	abdominal aortic aneurysm
AASV	anterior accessory saphenous vein
ABI	ankle/brachial pressure index
ACA	anterior cerebral artery
ACoA	anterior communicating artery
AI	acceleration index
AICA	anterior inferior cerebellar artery
ALARA	as low as reasonably achievable
AT	acceleration time
ATA	anterior tibial artery
ATCV	anterior thigh circumflex vein
ATV	anterior tibial vein
AV	arteriovenous
CCA	common carotid artery
CEA	carotid endarterectomy
CFA	common femoral artery
CFV	common femoral vein
CIA	common iliac artery
CIV	common iliac vein
CTA	computed tomographic angiography
CW	continuous-wave [Doppler]
DGC	depth gain compensation
DSA	digital subtraction angiography
DVT	deep vein thrombosis
ECA	external carotid artery
EDR	end diastolic ratio

EDV	end diastolic velocity
EIA	external iliac artery
EIV	external iliac vein
ESP	early systolic peak
EVAR	endovascular aneurysm repair
FN	false negative
FP	false positive
FV	femoral vein
GSV	great saphenous vein
HITS	high-intensity transient signals
ICA	internal carotid artery
IIA	internal iliac artery
IIV	internal iliac vein
IMA	inferior mesenteric artery
IMV	inferior mesenteric vein
IVC	inferior vena cava
IVUS	intravascular ultrasound
KE	kinetic energy
LIMA	left internal mammary artery
MCA	middle cerebral artery
MRA	magnetic resonance angiography
PAS	peripheral access system
PASV	posterior accessory saphenous vein
PCA	posterior cerebral artery
PCoA	posterior communicating artery
PE	potential energy
PE	pulmonary embolism
PFA	profunda femoris artery
PFV	profunda femoris vein
PI	pulsatility index
PICA	posterior inferior cerebellar artery
PICC	peripherally inserted central catheters
PPG	photoplethysmography
PRF	pulse repetition frequency
PSA	persistent sciatic artery
PSB	pansystolic spectral broadening
PSV	peak systolic velocity

PTA	posterior tibial artery
PTCV	posterior thigh circumflex vein
PTFE	polytetrafluoroethylene
PTV	posterior tibial veins
RAR	renal–aortic ratio
RI	resistance index
RIMA	right internal mammary artery
ROC	receiver operating characteristics
SFA	superficial femoral artery
SFj	saphenofemoral junction
SFV	superficial femoral vein
SMA	superior mesenteric artery
SMC	smooth muscle cell
SMV	superior mesenteric vein
SPj	saphenopopliteal junction
SSV	small saphenous vein
SVC	superior vena cava
TCCD	transcranial colour Doppler
TCD	transcranial Doppler
TE	thigh extension of SSV
TGC	time gain compensation
TIA	transient ischaemic attack
TIPS	transjugular intrahepatic portosystemic shunting
TN	true negative
TOS	thoracic outlet syndrome
TP	true positive
TSC	time sensitivity control
UGS	ultrasound-guided sclerotherapy

PRINCIPLES OF VASCULAR ULTRASOUND

Vascular ultrasound combines various modalities to study blood vessels and blood flow (Fig. 1.1). Modern systems use B-mode and pulsed Doppler combined as the duplex scanner. This book will not attempt to explore all aspects of ultrasound physics as they are covered in dedicated texts listed at the end of the book as 'Recommended reading'. However, vascular ultrasound cannot be understood without discussing basic principles.

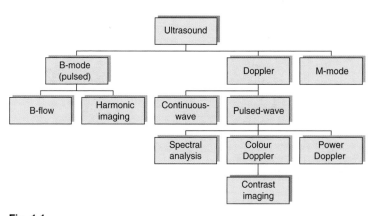

Fig. 1.1

Modalities used in vascular ultrasound to study blood vessels and blood flow

BASIC ULTRASOUND PRINCIPLES

Basic characteristics of sound waves are outlined in Box 1.1.

Box 1.1: Characteristics of sound waves
- **Frequency**: number of cycles per second (1 Hz = 1 cycle/s)
- **Period**: time for one cycle (seconds)
- **Wavelength**: length of one cycle (mm)
- **Velocity**: speed of sound wave propagation (cm/s)
- **Amplitude**: amount of energy in a sound wave.
- **Power**: rate of energy transfer (W)
- **Intensity**: power/area (W/m^2)

Ultrasound has a frequency >20 KHz, outside the range of human hearing. Frequencies used are millions of cycles per second (MHz). Ultrasound is generated and detected by mechanical oscillations from synthetic piezo-electric crystals (piezo-pressure) (Fig. 1.2).

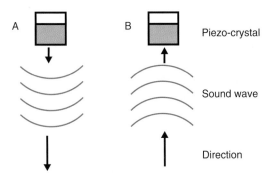

Fig. 1.2

Ultrasound signals

A: An alternating current applied to a piezo-crystal causes it to expand and contract to generate ultrasound at the same frequency that passes into the body.

B: Reflected sound waves strike a crystal and produce alternating electrical signals at the same frequency that are then processed by the ultrasound machine.

Passage of ultrasound through tissues

Ultrasound interacts with tissues as it propagates and returns (Fig. 1.3); properties are shown in Box 1.2.

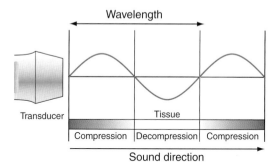

Fig. 1.3

Passage of ultrasound through tissues

Ultrasound travels as a longitudinal wave that causes tissue particles to oscillate in the same direction and at the same frequency.

Box 1.2: Properties of ultrasound

- **Propagation velocity**: average in soft tissue = 1540 m/s
- **Acoustic impedance**: resistance to transmission through a tissue – average in soft tissue = 1.6 kg/m^2/s (Rayls)
- **Interface**: junction between tissues of different acoustic impedances
- **Reflection**: when ultrasound strikes an interface larger than the wavelength at angles approaching 90° (Fig. 1.4)
- **Refraction**: when ultrasound strikes an interface beyond a critical angle away from 90° (Fig. 1.5)
- **Scattering**: as ultrasound strikes particles or a rough surface (Fig. 1.6)
- **Interference**: several sound waves with different frequencies pass through a tissue and enhance or compete with each other
- **Attenuation**: loss of ultrasound energy as it passes through tissues, proportional to the ultrasound frequency, distance from the transducer to the study site, and tissue density (Fig. 1.7)
- **Absorption**: conversion of ultrasound energy to heat as it travels through tissues

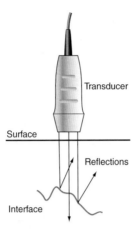

Fig. 1.4

Reflection

A 'strong reflector' is one where impedances on each side of the interface are considerably different.

- Most soft tissues: only 1–2 per cent reflected.
- Soft tissue and air: >99 per cent reflected so that coupling gel is required between transducer and skin.
- Soft tissue and bone: ≈40 per cent reflected so that transcranial studies can be difficult.
- Reflections from blood are weak compared with those from solid tissues.

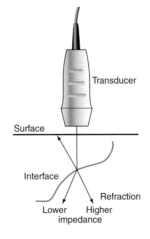

Fig. 1.5

Refraction

Part of the beam is reflected and the remainder continues to be transmitted but at a different angle depending on the velocity differences for each medium.

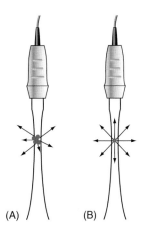

Fig. 1.6

Scattering

This occurs when ultrasound strikes a particle or object which is the same size or smaller than the ultrasound wavelength.

A: A particle approximately the same size as the wavelength scatters the wave to a variable degree in different directions. The degree of scattering depends on the ultrasound frequency and angle of insonation.

B: A particle smaller than the wavelength such as a red blood cell scatters the wave to an equal degree in all directions (termed **Rayleigh scattering**; Baron John William Rayleigh (1842–1919), an English physicist) independent of the angle of insonation.

(A)   (B)

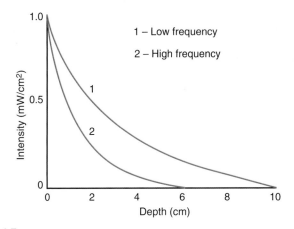

Fig. 1.7

Attenuation

- Exponential decay, mostly from absorption but also from reflection, refraction, scattering and diffraction.
- Less for low-frequency signals, as used for deep abdominal scanning.
- Greater for high-frequency signals, as used for superficial scanning.
- Low for blood, higher for soft tissues, and very high for lung and bone.

The Doppler effect: interaction of ultrasound with flowing blood

If a source is emitting sound waves, the frequency of reflected sound from an object in its path increases or decreases if the object is moving towards or away from the source respectively. This is the **Doppler effect** (Christian Andreas Doppler (1803–1863), an Austrian mathematician) and the change in frequency is the **Doppler shift**. Ultrasound from a stationary probe directed towards flowing blood detects a Doppler shift from red blood cells that is proportional to blood flow velocity and well within the audible range (Fig. 1.8).

The Doppler shift (f_d) is calculated as:

$$f_d = \frac{2 f_o v \cos \theta}{c}$$

where:

f_o = ultrasound frequency transmitted from the probe

v = velocity of moving blood

θ = angle between the direction of blood flow and axis of insonation

c = velocity of ultrasound in tissue (1540 m/s)

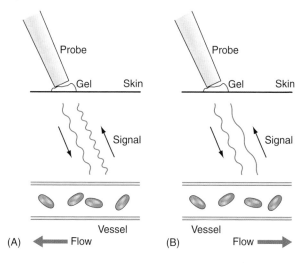

Fig. 1.8

Doppler shift

A: Blood moving towards the probe produces a positive Doppler shift.

B: Blood moving away from the probe produces a negative Doppler shift.

For example, if:

$$f_o = 5f_o \times 10^6 \ (5\,\text{MHz})$$
$$v = 100\,\text{cm/s}$$
$$\theta = 60°, \text{ so } \cos\theta = 0.5$$
$$f_d = (2 \times 5 \times 10^6 \times 100 \times 0.5)/1540 = 3246 \text{ cycles/s} \approx 3.2\,\text{KHz}$$

The blood flow velocity (v) is calculated from the Doppler shift as:

$$v = f_d c/2f_o \cos\theta$$

For example, if:

$$f_d = 5000 \text{ cycles/s} = 5.0\,\text{KHz}$$
$$f_o = 7.5 \times 106 \ (7.5\,\text{MHz})$$
$$\theta = 60°, \text{ so } \cos\theta = 0.5$$
$$v = (5000 \times 1540)/(2 \times 7.5 \times 10^6 \times 0.5) = 1.027\,\text{m/s} \approx 100\,\text{cm/s}$$

Ultrasound machines calculate Doppler shifts for any incident angle. Theoretically, if $\theta = 90°$ then $\cos\theta = 0$ and no flow signal will register. An error in measuring θ causes larger errors in velocity calculation as θ increases and it is best to avoid $\theta > 60°$. For example:

a 5 per cent error for $\theta = 30°$ results in a 5 per cent error for velocity, whereas

a 5 per cent error for $\theta = 70°$ results in a 20 per cent error for velocity.

TRANSDUCERS AND THE ULTRASOUND BEAM

Continuous-wave probes

A pencil probe contains two piezo-crystals, one to send and the other to receive signals (Fig. 1.9). The probe usually has air backing for greater sensitivity. It operates at only one continuous frequency, the optimum being around 8 MHz.

Pulsed-wave transducers

Modern pulsed-wave transducers are constructed with a backing to the piezo-crystals to dampen resonance (Fig. 1.10) with a row of piezo-crystal elements known as the 'array'.

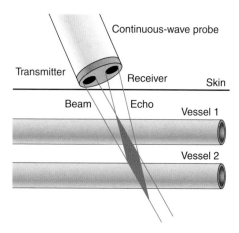

Fig. 1.9

The probe for continuous-wave Doppler

The dark-shaded segment represents the area of maximum sensitivity to receive the signal and covers multiple vessels in the field.

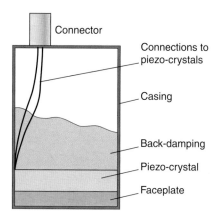

Fig. 1.10

Pulsed-wave transducer design

- Faceplate in front to prevent reflection.
- Back-damping layer behind to reduce oscillations.

Transducer characteristics are the:

- **footprint**: shape of the transducer surface
- **field of view**: area covered by the beam
- **dimensions**: shape of the transducer in three dimensions
  - **length**: the elevation plane
  - **width**: the plane of array or scan plane
  - **thickness**: determines the frequency.

The pulsed ultrasound beam

The main beam is three-dimensional and projected in a certain direction. Other lower intensity beams with the same frequency are produced (Fig. 1.11). Interactions between the numerous different components that make up a sound wave are termed **side lobes** and are three-dimensional in the array and elevation planes. Interference between the many waves from multiple piezo-crystals in an array causes **grating lobes** which are two-dimensional only in the plane of the array.

Each reflected echo that returns to the transducer is represented by a pixel assigned brightness or colour depending on the ultrasound mode. Many pixels together make an image. Piezo-crystals for pulsed ultrasound have an inherent resonant frequency but modern transducers use broad-band piezo-crystals that generate variable frequencies. This allows different modes to appear to be operating simultaneously.

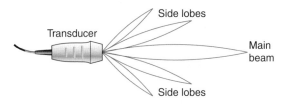

Fig. 1.11
Main beam and side lobes

Image quality is determined by:

- **pulse repetition frequency** (PRF): the frequency for emitting pulses from the transducer (KHz)
- **depth of view**: this depends on the ultrasound frequency, power of the signals and tissue type
- **time gain compensation** (TGC): echoes from numerous depths can be suppressed or enhanced, particularly for otherwise attenuated deeper signals, to provide even brightness throughout the depth of view
- **dynamic range**: allows the operator to increase or reduce the range of echo brightness levels processed. If the dynamic range is reduced (compression increased), lower-level echoes are suppressed allowing greater contrast of higher intensity signals. This is a pre-processing function so that if low-level echoes are to be examined then the area must be re-imaged with a higher dynamic range
- **compression curves**: manipulate the way in which echo brightness is stored and assigned shades of grey on the display. This is a post-processing function so that the image does not have to be rescanned
- **field of view and lines of sight**: the extent of image displayed on the screen and number of lines composing the image
- **frame rate**: the image is erased when the process has completed a field of view, and the screen is refreshed with a new image. This frame rate is set to produce what appears to be continuous real-time scanning. The display can be frozen at any time
- **persistence**: averages the brightness or colour allocated to each pixel over more than one frame. Increased persistence smooths the appearance of real-time images. The apparent frame rate is slowed even though the actual frame rate remains unchanged. However, this reduces temporal resolution.

Beam focusing and steering

An ultrasound beam is focused to a **focal point** where the beam intensity is maximal, after which it diverges to a progressively larger diameter and lower intensity (Fig. 1.12).

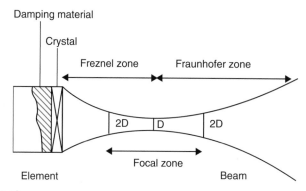

Fig. 1.12

A focused ultrasound beam

- Near field (Fresnel zone) between the source and focal point.
- Focal point (D) where the beam becomes smallest in diameter.
- Focal zone over which the width is less than twice the minimum width at the focal point (2D).
- Far field (Fraunhofer zone) beyond the focal point.

The ultrasound beam in the elevation plane is focused by an acoustic lens and this is not adjustable. The beam is also focused in the array plane and this can be controlled. Electronic focusing varies the sequence for activating piezo-crystals in the array. Selected piezo-crystals grouped within the array act as a single but larger element. Each is pulsed at different times to steer and/or focus ultrasound wave-fronts (Fig. 1.13). The greater the number of crystals used, the better the beam shape is controlled. The longer the time delays between excitations of the elements, the greater the angle of steering.

Resolution

- **Axial resolution** is the ability to resolve two echoes along a beam. It is improved by short pulses at high frequencies.
- **Lateral resolution** is the ability to resolve two echoes across a beam. It is improved by electronic focusing with array transducers.
- **Temporal resolution** is the ability to resolve events at different times. It is improved by a high frame rate. With modern machines, it is rarely a problem for B-mode but it can be slow for colour and power Doppler.

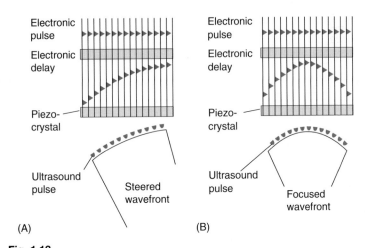

Fig. 1.13

Beam control

A: Excitation of elements on the left side before the right **steers** the beam outwards to the right.

B: Excitation of outer elements before the central elements **focuses** the beam forwards.

Types of array transducers

There are three types of electronic array transducers commonly used for vascular ultrasound. Operating frequencies are different for various manufacturers.

Linear array transducers (Fig. 1.14)

Characteristics are:

● **footprint**: straight row of 128–512 elements
● **field of view and lines of sight**: rectangular with parallel lines of sight
● **resolution**: even throughout depth due to parallel lines of sight
● **angle of insonation**: perpendicular to the transducer for B-mode and at 15° for Doppler to keep the signals independent

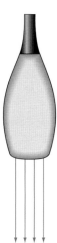

Fig. 1.14
Beam from a linear array transducer

- **beam production**: it never involves the entire array at any one time as the elements are excited in sequence
- **frequencies**: medium to high (5–12 MHz) to provide good superficial resolution though poor penetration so as to be favoured for superficial studies
- **steering**: possible with some machines
- **focusing**: possible.

Curvilinear (curved) array transducers (Fig. 1.15)
Characteristics are:

- **footprint**: long curved row of 128–512 piezo-elements
- **field of view and lines of sight**: larger field of view than for linear array transducers because of radial lines of sight but this makes angling more difficult
- **resolution**: decreased resolution at the edges of the field of view due to decreased numbers of elements forming the beam, and worse resolution in the deeper field of view due to diverging lines of sight. Resolution is poorer than for a linear array transducer but better than for a phased array transducer

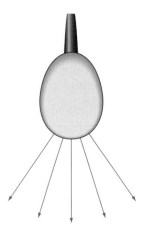

Fig. 1.15
Beam from a curved array transducer

- **angle of insonation:** perpendicular to the transducer for both B-mode and Doppler
- **beam production:** same as for the linear transducer
- **frequencies:** low to medium (2–7 MHz) so as to be used for deep studies
- **steering:** not possible
- **focusing:** possible.

Phased array transducers (Fig. 1.16)

Characteristics are:

- **footprint:** small with a short straight row of 64–128 piezo-crystals. This makes it easy to manoeuvre in tight locations, such as for transcranial studies, or where angling is difficult in the abdomen
- **field of view and lines of sight:** larger field of view than for linear array transducers because of radial lines of sight
- **resolution:** decreased resolution at the edges of the field of view due to smaller numbers of elements forming the beam; worse resolution in the deeper field of view due to radial lines of sight
- **angle of insonation:** radiating from the centre of the transducer for both B-mode and Doppler

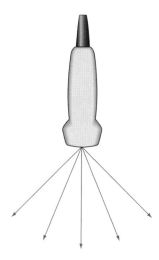

Fig. 1.16
Beam from a phased array transducer

- **frequencies**: lower than for the other transducers (2–4 MHz), providing good penetration for deep vessels
- **steering and beam production**: electronic throughout the field of view with all elements within the array used together to form a single group for B-mode, and separate elements steered to collect all Doppler shifts
- **focusing**: possible.

CONTINUOUS-WAVE (CW) DOPPLER

CW is the most simple Doppler mode. It is used to detect flow in peripheral arteries, for example during pressure studies, or to assess venous reflux. CW analyses many returning signals from several vessels in the line of sight of the beam so that it has no range or depth information. The operator must distinguish veins and arteries by flow characteristics alone as it provides only qualitative information.

Machine design (Fig. 1.17)
- The oscillator produces continuous-wave signals.
- The transmitter passes signals to the probe.

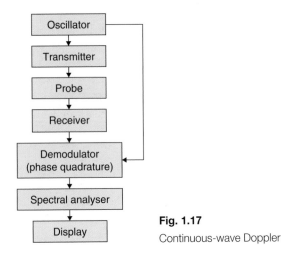

Fig. 1.17
Continuous-wave Doppler

● **The receiver** detects returning signals.
● **The demodulator** filters out returning signals with a frequency identical to the transmitted frequency leaving only the Doppler shift.
● **Phase quadrature** determines whether returning frequencies are greater or less than the emitted frequency to show whether flow is positive or negative.
● **The spectral analyser** processes all shifts within the signal. Fast Fourier transform establishes the frequency components.
● **The output** may be through a TV screen, recorder or audio system.

DUPLEX ULTRASOUND SCANNING

Most modern machines combine two modalities that use pulsed ultrasound:

● **B-mode** (brightness)
● **pulsed-Doppler**.

The same transducer is used for each modality. The machine can switch between them at great speed to give an illusion of real-time imaging for each. Lower frequencies are required for Doppler than B-mode because reflectors from blood cells for Doppler are weaker than tissue echoes at the same depth.

Pulsed Doppler can then be viewed as either:

- **spectral Doppler** or
- **colour Doppler.**

The mode for spectral Doppler has a **gate** to provide a **sample volume** that can be placed precisely into any selected area in the B-mode image. The mode for colour Doppler has a **colour box** that can be changed in size or direction in the B-mode image.

B-mode ultrasound

B-mode provides two-dimensional, real-time, greyscale images (Fig. 5.6, page 84). As a beam sweeps through tissues, an image is created from information for the different lines of sight. This relates to the depth, direction and brightness of each echo.

Echogenicity

Echogenicity is the greyscale level assigned to each pixel and represents the acoustic impedance mismatch at interfaces. Greyscale echoes range from bright to dark according to the amount of reflection. A structure that returns echoes is **echoic** and if no echoes are returned then the area is **anechoic**. A strong reflector is represented as being bright and is **hyperechoic** and a weak reflector is shown as being dark or **hypoechoic**. An area in the image that shows reflections is referred to as **echogenic** and an area that shows no or weak reflections is **echolucent**. A structure that has a relatively uniform echogenicity is referred to as **homogeneous**, whether it be echogenic or echolucent, and a structure with variable echogenicity is referred to as **heterogeneous**, containing both echogenic and echolucent areas or echoes of varying brightness.

Tissue characteristics that affect echogenicity are:

- reflection and scattering at acoustic interfaces
- attenuation and absorption
- depth of the reflector.

Technical considerations that determine echogenicity are the:

- gain setting with a linear relation between gain and image brightness

- transducer frequency with high frequencies reducing echogenicity
- TGC settings
- dynamic range.

New techniques to improve resolution with B-mode have been made possible by increased computing capacity. Groups of pixels can be processed prior to display to reduce artefacts and enhance the image. Multiple lines of sight from different angles can be used to provide computed tomography that again markedly reduces various artefacts so as to further improve image quality.

Machine design (Fig. 1.18)

- **The pulse generator** produces very short electrical pulses for best resolution.
- **The beam tracker** determines the direction and shape of the beam.
- **The amplifier** increases the intensity of low level signals.
- **The demodulator** converts negative components from the signals to positive ones and processes all positive components.
- **The scan converter** manipulates data and stores digital signals to render them suitable for display.
- **The image** display is on a conventional TV monitor.

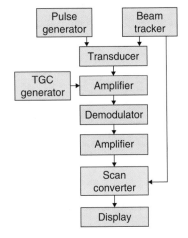

Fig. 1.18

B-mode ultrasound

Artefacts for B-mode scanning

Obtaining an ideal B-mode image assumes that sound travels at a constant speed in a straight line, attenuation is uniform, and echoes return directly to the transducer from the central axis of the beam. In practice, these are difficult to achieve, predisposing to artefacts.

Image displacement

- **Mirror artefacts** occur at high impedance mismatch specular interfaces. A structure closer to the transducer than the interface is directly insonated by the beam, giving an image in its true position. The beam continues on and is then reflected from the interface to re-insonate the original structure. This produces a second image of the structure which is seen at a corresponding distance on the other side of the 'mirror' to its true position. This most commonly occurs at the pleura–lung interface, duplicating subclavian and internal mammary vessels and the hepatic veins.
- **Reverberation artefacts** are multiple false images of the same interface at different depths. They are caused by repeated reflections between two high impedance mismatch interfaces. Some energy returns to the transducer at each reverberation.
- **Comet tail artefacts** are a form of reverberation with echoes decreasing in brightness and width as depth increases.
- **Ringdown artefacts** result from resonance when an ultrasound beam strikes a group of air bubbles (Fig.16.2, page 314). Very little energy is lost so that there is no decrease in brightness of the artefact with increasing depth.
- **Side lobes** and **grating lobes** produce echoes that are attributed to the central axis of the main beam.
- **Beam width** and **slice thickness artefacts** result from echoes that are produced by any part of the beam being attributed to the central axis, producing images to one side of the true position. Low frequencies result in increased beam width and slice thickness.
- **Velocity artefacts** occur when the ultrasound velocity varies in different insonated tissues causing error in the calculated depth of the image.
- **Depth** or **range ambiguity** can occur if the PRF is increased. At a high PRF, a pulse may be emitted before the signal from the

previous pulse has returned, and both are interpreted as being associated. The image built up from the multiple echoes appears to be somewhere between the transducer and the real structure.

Image loss

- **Acoustic shadowing** results from total reflection from bone, bowel gas or a calcified arterial plaque (Fig. 5.6D, page 85). The reflecting object must be wider than the beam width to cause shadowing.
- **Edge shadowing** results from dropout of lines of sight due to reflection and refraction at the edges of round structures (Fig. 2.1, page 34).
- **Loss of spatial resolution** can occur if the voltage in the elements is not uniform, or if returning echoes fail to strike the aperture at the same time.
- **Dropout** occurs deep to relatively highly attenuating tissue. Dropout can be produced by setting the TGC too low at a particular level, or if there is an incorrect transmitting frequency or inadequate output power.

Image enhancement

Acoustic enhancement causing apparent increased echogenicity can occur deep to a structure of low attenuation, or if the TGC is set too high at a particular level giving a false image of increased brightness.

Spectral Doppler

Ultrasound is emitted in pulses similar to B-mode, and a gate is used to determine the interval after emission when returning signals are received, and therefore the depth from which the sample is taken. Spectral analysis shows the Doppler shift spectrum and direction, usually displayed as the maximum velocity rather than frequency (Fig. 4.14, page 72). To calculate spectral Doppler shifts takes 64–128 pulses per scan line. The information is quantitative.

The maximum possible PRF and maximum recordable Doppler shift are dependent on the sample depth, since the next ultrasound pulse should not be emitted before all information from the previous pulse is received. The upper limit for the Doppler shift that can be measured without range ambiguity is the **Nyquist limit** $\leq$ PRF/2 – otherwise echoes would be returning while signals are being transmitted. The period that the gate is open determines the axial region over which the sample is taken and this is the sample volume. Pulsed Doppler captures a far smaller range of frequencies than CW Doppler.

Machine design (Fig. 1.19)

This is similar to the design previously shown for CW Doppler, with the addition of a **PRF generator** or **clock**. The clock provides uniform transmitted pulses and its timing determines the depth and length of the sample volume.

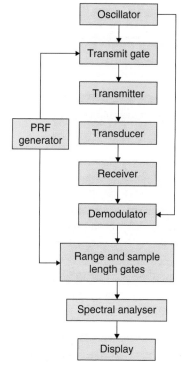

Fig. 1.19
Spectral Doppler

Artefacts for spectral Doppler

Aliasing

Aliasing or Doppler shift ambiguity can occur with pulsed Doppler if there is a high velocity at an arterial stenosis. If the Doppler shift exceeds the Nyquist limit, then high frequencies are 'wrapped around' and appear to be in the opposite direction relative to the baseline (Fig. 1.20).

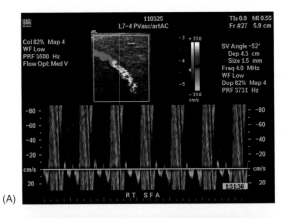

(A)

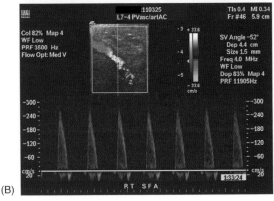

(B)

Fig. 1.20

Aliasing shown by spectral Doppler

A: Aliasing is easily recognized as the peak is shown in the opposite direction.

B: Increasing the velocity scale eliminates aliasing to restore a complete signal.

From the Doppler equation:

$$f_{max} = 2f_0 v_{max} \cos \theta / c = \text{PRF}/2 \text{ so that}$$
$$v_{max} = c\text{PRF} / 4f_0 \cos \theta$$

This shows that the ways to reduce aliasing with pulsed-Doppler are to:

- increase the velocity scale (PRF)
- reduce the transmitted frequency f_0
- increase the angle of insonation θ (decrease $\cos\theta$), or
- move the baseline.

Modern machines use an automated technique to avoid aliasing. Echoes can be received from two sample volume depths, the deeper one from the vessel of interest and the superficial one not in a vessel. The machine is programmed to sense that a pulse must be emitted and received before the next pulse is emitted. A high PRF is used to make it appear that the reflected signal comes from the more superficial sample even though the Doppler shift comes from the deeper sample (Fig. 13.7, page 280).

Movement and filter artefact

Pulsations of structures adjacent to blood vessels create high-intensity, low-frequency Doppler shifts that can swamp reflections from blood flow. This is prevented by high-pass filters, but setting the wall filter threshold too high can lead to loss of the diastolic part of the wave-form or loss of low flow signals altogether.

Periodic tissue motion artefact

Rapid periodic motion of solid tissue can result in horizontal bands in the spectral waveform.

Colour Doppler

Doppler shifts are determined from multiple sites within a specified **colour box**. Mean frequencies and flow directions are calculated and assigned colours displayed in real-time as an overlay on a B-mode image to show two-dimensional flow within vessels.

As with B-mode, many elements across the transducer face produce the colour profile. Typically, there are 8–20 pulses per line of sight to

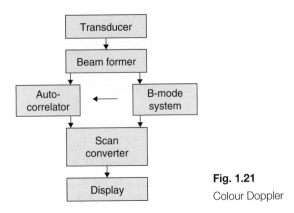

Fig. 1.21

Colour Doppler

obtain frequency shift information for each pixel, and this is termed the **ensemble length** or **packet size**. Frequency is calculated for each gate and assigned a colour on the screen. The pixel position corresponds to the site from where the echo originated. Colour is shown in terms of flow direction, mean Doppler shift, and variance around the mean. The information is qualitative.

Machine design (Fig. 1.21)

- The beam former determines the direction and shape of the beam.
- The autocorrelator compares successive echoes from each line of sight to detect change.
- The scan converter manipulates data and stores digital signals to render them suitable for display.
- The image display is on a conventional colour TV monitor.

Artefacts for colour Doppler

Aliasing

Aliasing affects each pixel in the colour box where velocities are higher than the Nyquist limit. This produces regions of reversed colour that can be confused with true reverse flow or turbulence (Fig. 1.22).

Mirror and twinkling artefacts

The principles for mirror artefacts are as described for B-mode artefacts (Fig. 1.23). Twinkling is noise created by multiple reflections

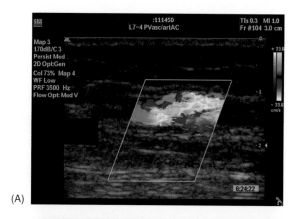

(A)

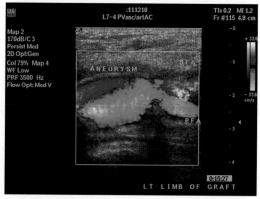

(B)

Fig. 1.22

Distinction of aliasing from true flow reversal with colour Doppler

A: Aliasing shows pale red and pale blue high-frequency colours without a dark line between as there is no phase of zero flow.

B: Flow reversal shows a fine dark line of demarcation between deep red and blue low-frequency colours.

(Fig. 1.24). These are corrected by reducing the Doppler gain or decreasing the angle of insonation.

Flash artefact

This occurs when there is sudden movement of tissue or the transducer causing Doppler shifts to register within the entire colour box.

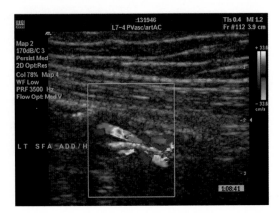

Fig. 1.23
Mirror artefact at a calcified arterial wall

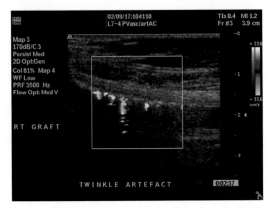

Fig. 1.24
Twinkle artefact from an arterial bypass graft wall

Periodic tissue motion artefact

This results from rapid periodic motion of solid tissue causing banding with colour Doppler.

Colour bleeding

This is when colour pixels appear in regions where there are no Doppler shifts due to setting the colour Doppler gain or colour write priority too high. It also occurs because colour pixel size is larger than B-mode pixel size.

POWER DOPPLER

In this mode, colour is assigned to the power of the Doppler signal rather than the Doppler frequency shift. Flow is usually displayed with one colour of varying brightness (Fig. 1.25). Power Doppler is used to detect very slow flow, flow in small vessels, or where transducer angling is awkward. Power Doppler can be used in conjunction with contrast agents.

Advantages

● The signal is not dependent on the angle of insonation, although there must be a Doppler shift.
● Aliasing does not occur with power Doppler since the power of the signal is independent of its apparent direction.
● The power of electronic noise is low so that the signal-to-noise ratio is improved, and a low PRF is used so that power Doppler is three to five times more sensitive to detecting low flow than colour Doppler, and is better able to define boundaries.

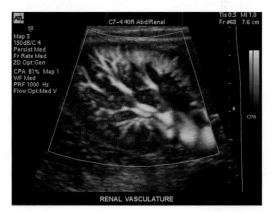

Fig. 1.25

Power Doppler image to show the renal hilar, interlobar and cortical arteries

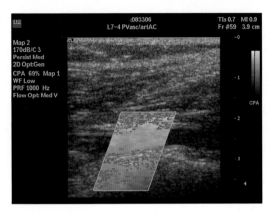

Fig. 1.26
Flash artefact with power Doppler

Limitations

- No directional information is provided so that adjacent vessels with flow in opposite directions appear the same, making it difficult to distinguish veins from arteries.
- There is a relatively low PRF so that there is poor temporal resolution.
- Due to the low PRF, power Doppler is particularly sensitive to flash artefact (Fig. 1.26).

TISSUE HARMONIC IMAGING

Tissue expands and compresses unevenly as ultrasound passes through, causing the waveform to produce frequencies that are multiples (harmonics) of the fundamental frequency. The B-mode beam-former transmits at one low frequency and the scan converter accepts only the higher harmonic frequencies. Harmonics travel only one way from tissue to transducer so that they are only attenuated by one passage. Harmonic echoes have extremely low amplitude and require advanced electronics to be recorded. Artefacts from superficial structures are reduced since these signals do not have sufficient energy to generate harmonics and are filtered out.

Pulse inversion harmonic imaging is another advance. Two pulses are transmitted, the first followed by a second which is identical but inverted. The two fundamental signals cancel and their two harmonic components reinforce to provide broader bandwidths with better resolution and sensitivity.

A combination of tissue harmonic imaging and power Doppler provides a very sensitive technique without the problem of aliasing so that a very low PRF can be used, allowing very low flow to be demonstrated.

CONTRAST IMAGING

Injected ultrasound contrast agents contain microbubbles that are non-linear reflectors or scatterers of ultrasound energy. When an ultrasound wave encounters a microbubble, it causes it to compress and expand in phase in the longitudinal direction just as for tissues. Microbubbles easily burst when they expand under insonation, generating considerable harmonic energy.

The colour Doppler system detects that Doppler shifts have occurred but it cannot assign the correct direction and velocity for flow. The image has a random mottled red and blue appearance that helps distinguish contrast from moving tissue. Power Doppler gives a more uniform appearance since it is non-directional. The technique can be used to detect almost stationary blood, such as trickle flow through a very tight arterial stenosis or flow in the microvasculature.

B-FLOW IMAGING

B-flow measures the amplitude of scatterers in flowing blood to provide an image that clearly shows the vessel lumen, a wide range of velocities, or plaque characteristics. Processing involves noise reduction and signal enhancement. B-flow imaging uses a higher frame rate and has better spatial resolution than colour Doppler. It is not subject to artefacts such as colour bleeding or aliasing. However, it cannot measure velocities or show flow direction.

2

PERFORMING A SCAN

Duplex ultrasound scans performed by well-trained practitioners are quick, relatively inexpensive, non-invasive and accurate. Investigation should be reserved for patients with reasonably severe disability or where a diagnosis is not clear. In many centres, duplex scanning has replaced arteriography as the initial investigation for patients being considered for operation.

CONTROLS FOR THE ULTRASOUND MACHINE

Settings and controls vary for different manufacturers but there is a common theme. Most have a preset menu for each anatomical site although some sonographers prefer to create their own settings. There are many adjustable controls (Boxes 2.1–2.6). Machines made by different manufacturers may have different names for the controls but they all serve the same purpose. Some machines do not have all of the functions listed while others have controls not mentioned here.

Box 2.1: Monitor controls and displays
- Brightness
- Contrast
- Colour velocity scale
- Patient annotation
- Mechanical and thermal indices
- Time gain compensation (TGC) curve
- Focal zones
- Depth scale
- Transducer frequency
- Colour and B-mode parameters

Box 2.2: Keyboard functions
- Annotations
- Transducer select key
- Setup select keys
- Function select keys
- Output/power
- Frame capture capabilities and cineloop
- Calculations: distances between objects, velocities and various ratios

Box 2.3: B-mode controls
- TGC/depth gain compensation (DGC)/time sensitivity control (TSC)
- Sector width
- Singular and multiple focal zones
- Depth of field of view
- Gain
- Pre- and post-processing zoom
- Dynamic range (compression curves)
- Greyscale maps
- B-mode chroma
- PRF
- Persistence/frame averaging/smoothing

Box 2.4: Controls for colour Doppler
- Baseline
- Echo-write priority (sensitivity/threshold)
- Frequency range
- Colour box position, size and angle
- Colour maps
- Wall filter
- Gain
- Colour invert
- Persistence/frame averaging/smoothing

Priority: when colour Doppler is activated, the control is set at a level that determines whether echoes with a brightness greater than the threshold are displayed only in B-mode while echoes with brightness less than the threshold are colour-coded. This helps to distinguish blood flow signals from tissue movement.

Box 2.5: Controls for spectral Doppler

- Baseline
- Velocity range (PRF control)
- Spectral invert
- Gain
- Sample volume size, position and angle
- Wall filter
- Sweep speed
- Doppler chroma

Box 2.6: Controls for power Doppler

- Baseline
- Echo-write priority/sensitivity/threshold
- Power box size, position and angle
- Power Doppler maps
- Wall filter
- Persistence

HOW TO OPTIMIZE THE IMAGE

It is usual practice to initially orientate anatomy and view pathology using **B-mode**, to proceed to qualitatively examine blood flow and flow abnormalities with **colour Doppler**, and then to quantitatively assess whether flow is normal or disturbed with **spectral Doppler**.

Box 2.7: Image orientation

Standardize how images are displayed in transverse and longitudinal views (Fig. 2.1, page 34). Use an orientation marker on the transducer and orientation icon on the image if it is present. Orientate yourself by using known landmarks.

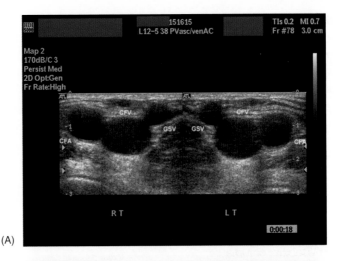

(A)

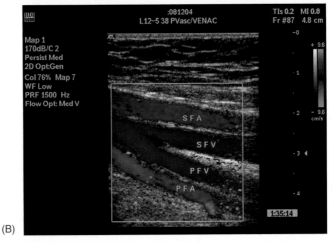

(B)

Fig. 2.1

Image orientation: personal practice

A: Transverse view: hold the transducer so that the patient's image is facing towards you. When scanning the saphenofemoral junction for the 'Mickey Mouse' sign, the medial aspect will be on the right of screen for the right lower limb and left of the screen for the left lower limb.

B: Longitudinal view: hold the transducer so that the cephalad end is to the left of the screen. When scanning femoral vessels, the common femoral is to the left of the screen and the femoral and profunda femoris vessels are to the right of the screen.

All modalities

- Select the appropriate transducer (see regional chapters).
- Apply copious gel.
- Avoid excessive transducer pressure.
- Select windows where vessels are most superficial.
- Find windows through soft tissues with uniform density and low acoustic impedance such as muscle, avoiding fat and strong reflectors such as gas or bone.
- Move the patient into different positions or take advantage of a tilt bed.
- Increase power as a last resort (ALARA: as low as reasonably achievable).

B-Mode

- Position the focal zone just deep to the area of interest. This decreases beam thickness and therefore improves lateral resolution at the level of interest.
- If possible, insonate vessels at 90° for maximum specular reflection and to give best definition of the vessel wall, atheromatous plaque or thrombus.
- To ensure correct gain, image a 'clear' section of lumen in longitudinal, increase gain until the lumen fills with noise, and then decrease gain until the lumen becomes clear of noise and black in appearance.
- Adjust TGC throughout the duration of the scan.
- Reduce the scanning depth to increase the frame rate and decrease signal attenuation.

Colour Doppler

- Increase the colour gain and echo-write priority to a level where there is good colour filling of vessels but no colour bleeding.
- Reduce the width of the colour box to increase the frame rate.
- Steer the colour box or 'heel and toe' the transducer to avoid insonating the vessel of interest at 90° otherwise Doppler shifts will not be coded.

- Change to a higher frequency transducer to increase Doppler shifts if low-velocity flow is suspected but cannot be colour-coded.

Spectral Doppler

- Set power and gain low and adjust levels up from the minimum until the optimum signal is achieved with the least surrounding background noise. This helps distinguish true spectral broadening from artefact.
- Initially, set the wall filter on minimum to ensure that low velocities are not omitted from the spectral trace.
- 'Heel and toe' the transducer to ensure that the Doppler angle is always ≤60°.
- Increase sample size when analysing low velocities to allow more time for Doppler shifts to be detected.
- Use 'micromovements' to ensure that the sample volume remains in the centre of the vessel.

Limitations

- Transducer pressure can block flow in veins.
- It can be difficult to obtain the best angle for insonation and Doppler sampling.
- The colour display is in two dimensions whereas flow is three-dimensional.
- The short time required to rapidly and repetitively switch from B-mode to spectral Doppler reduces the frame rate for B-mode and PRF for pulsed Doppler.
- The small sample size for spectral Doppler provides information only for a small segment in the larger field of view.
- The sample volume for spectral Doppler is shown on a frozen B-mode image but the signal will be reduced or lost if the transducer or patient moves. The Doppler shift displayed is also affected if the transducer's 'heel and toe' angle is changed after the image is frozen. These problems can be overcome by using B-mode and spectral Doppler in real-time.

- Displayed flow may be generated from different times within the cardiac cycle due to the time delays required to produce a complete colour image.
- Decreasing the range gate size improves axial resolution but decreases sensitivity owing to reduced signal-to-noise ratio.
- Decreasing the beam thickness reduces the transit time for red blood cells to cross the beam so that sampling time is decreased, causing uncertainty for Doppler shift readings.

Abdominal studies can be limited by:

- obesity that leads to loss of signal beyond a depth of 15–18 cm
- gas pockets in the stomach or bowel that produce acoustic shadows
- calcification and scar tissue from previous surgery causing shadowing or extensive beam attenuation
- tortuous vessels that can be hard to track making it difficult to obtain a Doppler angle <60°.

To avoid these problems:

- fast the patient
- turn the patient to right or left lateral decubitus and use a posterolateral window
- tilt the table at various angles to shift gas to different positions in the bowel
- use the transducer to massage the abdomen from lateral to medial to push bowel gas away
- use the small phased array transducer to avoid obstruction.

Tips!

- Apply reasonable pressure to the transducer to improve the image but not so much as to cause pain.
- Ask the patient to hold the breath while taking a Doppler sample – remember to tell the patient when to recommence breathing.

PERIPHERAL OR CAROTID ARTERIAL STUDIES

Machine settings for peripheral or carotid arteries

B-Mode

● Use the maximum dynamic range to aid plaque characterization.

Colour Doppler

● Set the colour velocity range to approximately +35 to −35 cm/s to highlight stenoses without spurious aliasing throughout the entire artery.
● Decrease the colour scale and increase colour gain to show low flow distal to an occlusion or high-grade stenosis.
● Choose a colour map that easily highlights high velocities.
● Use a low wall filter setting to ensure that low velocities are not filtered out. Increase the wall filter to prevent wall motion artefact when scanning carotid arteries that are highly mobile with respiration.

Spectral Doppler

● Set the velocity scale to +150 to −50 cm/s.
● Use a small sample volume to help clear up the spectral trace.
● Place the sample volume in the centre of the artery or within the stenotic jet stream.
● Decrease the spectral Doppler scale and increase spectral gain to show low flow distal to an occlusion or high-grade stenosis.
● Use a low wall filter to ensure that low velocities are not filtered out. Again increase the wall filter when interrogating highly mobile arteries.

Scanning techniques for peripheral and carotid arteries

● Scan in B-mode in longitudinal and transverse to fully assess the arteries and plaque type.
● Take each artery in turn and use colour Doppler to help identify the artery and highlight sites of increased velocities.

- Place spectral sample volumes to measure velocities at intervals along the artery, particularly proximal, within and distal to areas of aliasing.

Use **B-mode** to:

- locate arteries, stents and bypass grafts: these are easily differentiated from veins as they are mostly incompressible with transducer pressure
- orientate arterial pathology to appropriate bony or vascular landmarks
- study atheromatous plaque in transverse and longitudinal with the colour turned off to ensure correct characterization
- note the position and type of plaque, describe plaque morphology as homogeneous, heterogeneous or calcified, and describe surface characteristics as smooth, irregular or ulcerated
- measure diameters of arteries, aneurysms or grafts and look for tortuosity or ectasia.

Tip!

Use the adjacent vein as a guide if the artery is occluded.

Use **colour Doppler** to:

- help identify arteries and bypass grafts
- note flow direction
- indicate the presence, location and length of each arterial stenosis or occlusion
- highlight areas of maximum velocities by colour jets or colour aliasing to show the best place to position the sample volume for spectral Doppler
- identify atheromatous plaque that is not visible with B-mode from a corresponding blank area in the colour box (Fig. 5.6A, page 84)
- identify collaterals and their flow direction
- identify the residual lumen diameter of an aneurysm.

Use **spectral Doppler** to:

- conclusively differentiate between arteries and veins by analysis of flow direction and waveform morphology
- determine which artery is being studied by whether there is a low- or high-resistance signal according to the particular arterial bed
- obtain a spectral trace of velocities proximal to and at sites of stenoses and note whether spectral broadening is present or absent to help determine the severity of stenosis
- 'walk' the Doppler sample volume through a stenosis and use 'micromovements' from side to side to ensure that the sample volume is in the centre of the artery or jet stream, and that the highest velocities are obtained
- indicate proximal or distal disease from waveform analysis
- calculate appropriate ratios
- document the exact length and location of arterial stenoses and occlusions.

Opinion!

If there is a stenosis with an eccentric jet stream, place the cursor parallel to the actual flow direction shown by colour Doppler and not parallel to the vessel wall (Fig. 6.7, page 107).

PERIPHERAL VENOUS STUDIES

Machine settings for venous reflux and thrombosis

B-Mode

- Use low gain and power to prevent oversaturation of surrounding tissues or artefact within the vessel.
- High gain will cause thrombus to appear highly echogenic, while low gain will better show low echogenicity,
- Use a high contrast setting (low dynamic range) to highlight the vein walls when testing for vein compression or venous reflux.

● Use a low contrast setting (high dynamic range) to view thrombus and surrounding tissue.

Colour Doppler

● Set a low colour velocity range of $+10$ to -10 cm/s but increase the range if this produces unacceptably high colour artefact or reduces the frame rate too much.
● Select a relatively even colour hue across the frequency range as velocity information and aliasing are not used to test for venous disease.
● Optimize colour gain and priority settings to allow good colour filling without bleeding.

Spectral Doppler

● Set the velocity range to $+100$ to -100 cm/s when testing for reflux and $+50$ to -50 cm/s when testing for venous thrombosis. These ranges can be reduced for low flow states.
● Set the wall filter to a minimum so that low flow traces are not filtered out.
● Open the sample volume to obtain as much information from the vessel as possible.
● Set the Doppler display sweep to the slowest speed to easily identify flow patterns.

Scanning techniques for peripheral venous studies

Venous scanning has less emphasis on spectral Doppler and more on B-mode and colour Doppler. The sample volume does not need to be steered absolutely parallel to the vein wall.

Use **B-mode** to:

● locate veins and map their course and connections
● identify perforators passing through the deep fascia
● measure diameters of incompetent saphenous junctions and refluxing saphenous veins and perforators
● assess whether veins can be compressed or contain visible thrombus
● classify the age of thrombus.

Use **colour Doppler** to:

● distinguish veins from arteries
● show the direction of venous flow and indicate the presence of reflux
● determine whether the vein is patent, partially or fully thrombosed
● identify collaterals.

Use **spectral Doppler** to:

● confirm venous occlusions
● confirm colour Doppler directional information
● quantify duration of reverse flow to categorize reflux.

Scanning techniques for venous flow and reflux

Scan with the limbs dependent to fill with blood, either standing or on a tilt table feet down in reverse Trendelenburg (Friedrich Trendelenburg (1844–1924), a German surgeon).

● Take each vein in turn and identify it with B-mode in transverse.
● Then change to colour Doppler to test for reflux in longitudinal.
● Use spectral Doppler with the sample volume filling the vein if there is doubt about the duration of reverse flow with colour Doppler.
● Follow each vein along its full length with B-mode and periodically test for reflux with colour Doppler.
● Detect perforators in transverse and test for reflux with the perforator 'opened up'.
● Use spectral Doppler if the colour flow direction is ambiguous.

Scanning techniques for venous thrombosis

● Assess all veins for **compressibility** with B-mode in transverse. Use pressure from the transducer or counter-pressure from the other hand to assess compressibility.
● Test for **patency** with colour Doppler in longitudinal and transverse to ensure partial thrombus is not missed (Fig. 9.7, page 190). This may be confirmed by spectral Doppler.
● Test for each at 1–2 cm intervals along the vein or when there is B-mode evidence of thrombus.

● Use spectral Doppler to test for **phasicity** in proximal veins. Reduced or absent phasicity indicates thrombus proximal to the test site (Fig.11.20, page 245).

ABDOMINAL STUDIES

Machine settings for abdominal studies

Use high gain settings for all modalities because of the depth of most vessels. However, high gain degrades spatial resolution so that there is a loss of contrast resolution if the signal is 'overgained'.

B-Mode

● Use a high dynamic range (low contrast) to help visualize pathology such as mural thrombus in an aneurysm.
● Decrease sector width to increase the frame rate.
● Use only a single focal zone, as multiple focal zones decrease the frame rate giving a blurred appearance.

Colour Doppler

● Decrease the colour box width to increase the frame rate.
● Use a medium to high wall filter as the abdomen moves with respiration causing wall motion artefact.
● Set the colour velocity range to approximately $+35$ to -35 cm/s to highlight arterial stenoses without spurious aliasing, or $+10$ to -10 cm/s for venous studies.
● Make sure that the beam is not approaching at too large an angle and that the velocity range and wall filter settings are not too high if a vessel can be seen but no flow is detected.

Spectral Doppler

● Increase the sweep speed when studying renal arteries as this allows better identification of waveform parameters required for criteria ratios.
● Set the velocity scale to $+150$ to -50 cm/s for arterial studies and $+100$ to -100 cm/s for venous studies. These ranges can be reduced for low flow states.
● Use a medium wall filter.

Scanning techniques for abdominal vessels

Arterial examinations are identical to those in the periphery. However, there are some differences for venous studies. Scan with the patient supine or on a tilt table feet down in reverse Trendelenburg to allow viscera to drop down towards the pelvis away from the upper abdomen.

It is difficult to compress abdominal veins. Use colour Doppler to follow the veins, as loss of colour flow may suggest occlusive thrombus. Sample a spectral signal from a vein to confirm loss of flow. If flow is seen throughout the veins then they are patent although they could still be partially thrombosed. The age of a thrombus is difficult to define.

Abdominal venous reflux can be elicited by upper abdominal compression and arrested by lower abdominal compression. Ovarian vein reflux is usually spontaneous. It is difficult to produce intra-abdominal reflux by the Valsalva manoeuvre or distal limb compression.

3

SETTING UP A VASCULAR DIAGNOSTIC SERVICE

It is important to care for the interests of patients and sonographers. The reward for having the best equipment and working environment is improved productivity. Much can be done to lessen the risks of occupation-induced musculoskeletal injuries to vascular sonographers.

Much of this chapter is based on the Australasian Society for Ultrasound in Medicine's *Guidelines for Reducing Injuries to Sonographers and Sonologists*, prepared by Val Gregory and Cheryl Bass.

UNIT PREMISES

The configuration should be flexible and versatile.

Examination room

The examination room should:

- be close to the waiting room, patient facilities and processing areas
- be large enough to allow the ultrasound unit to be easily moved into position and provide an ergonomic couch position
- be able to be set up for opposite (usually left handed) scanning
- have flooring that allows easy movement of the ultrasound unit
- have adequate ventilation for the ultrasound unit, patient and staff

- have dimmable lighting
- have hand-washing facilities.

Environment

There should be:

- transducer-cleaning facilities
- a fume cupboard, ventilated container or self-filtering system if transducers are cleaned with noxious chemicals
- an emergency policy to manage spills if noxious chemicals are used.

PERSONNEL

A medical director and supervising sonographer with appropriate qualifications and experience are necessary, with other sonographers, clerical, nursing and research staff as required.

The medical director in conjunction with the supervising sonographer is responsible for:

- practice management
- rostering
- supervision of bookings
- patient management
- sonographer training
- safe equipment and a safe work environment
- equipment maintenance and operation
- patient and sonographer health and safety
- reporting.

For student sonographers, a senior sonographer should be available at all times and participate to a degree dependent on the student's competence and experience.

ULTRASOUND EQUIPMENT

The equipment chosen for a service depends on its particular interests and budget. Most manufacturers appreciate the need for ergonomic design. Costs should allow for the base unit, range of transducers required, upgrade options, a maintenance contract and warranty agreement. A system for regular equipment maintenance should include electrical safety checks, calibration and quality assurance. Components may include video storage and a hard copy printer.

Ultrasound machine

The ultrasound machine should:

● be modern equipment with good ergonomic design
● be fully adjustable to suit all staff and procedures
● be manoeuvrable with accessible, lockable wheels
● have easily accessible recording devices
● have a footrest
● have height-adjustable handles to enable sonographers to push the machine at the correct height for their body habitus.

Keyboard

The keyboard should:

● be height-adjustable
● be able to be rotated
● be user-friendly with frequently used functions most accessible. Some units have preset programs that allow keys to have multiple functions depending on the examination
● have space underneath to allow room for the sonographer's knees.

Monitor

The monitor should:

● have high definition to reduce flicker, improve image quality and lessen eye fatigue
● be height- and tilt-adjustable with lateral movement across the unit to reduce the need to reach and twist
● have accessible controls and locks.

Transducers

Transducers should:

● be large enough to allow a power (palmar) grip rather than a pinch grip

- be slip-resistant to assist grip
- be easy to change with lightweight cables and easy-to-access cable supports
- have cables long enough to permit unrestricted use
- be easily accessible.

Couch

The couch should:

- be height-adjustable and tiltable and able to go low enough to allow patients to get on and off unassisted
- be movable with wheels that are lockable and easy to release
- have 'uncluttered' sides and ends to allow sonographers to place their knees and feet underneath
- have a covering made of a material that allows easy cleaning
- be narrow enough so that the sonographer does not have to reach any further than necessary
- have an adjustable headrest and patient restraints if appropriate
- have electronic foot pedal controls that are accessible and easy to use.

Chair

The chair should:

- be mobile, height- and tilt-adjustable to suit all staff and procedures
- have back and thigh support and a footrest. A flat, gas-lift stool is an acceptable alternative
- be able to swivel so that the sonographer can rotate from the patient to the ultrasound machine keeping the posture aligned.

Accessories

Accessories needed are:

- gel bottles with large openings to reduce the strength needed to squeeze them
- a cushion to support the arm in abduction
- easy to reach gel wipes

- items such as support pads for the patient and sonographer
- gel bottle holders and linen that are easily accessible
- contaminated waste and sharps disposal containers for interventional procedures.

GUIDELINES FOR REDUCING INJURIES TO SONOGRAPHERS AND SONOLOGISTS

Some examinations force sonographers to work in awkward positions. Musculoskeletal injuries caused by repetitive scanning are often not apparent until the end of the day or at night. Injuries often take a long time to manifest and resolve. The severity of acute injury may be exacerbated by an existing chronic musculoskeletal injury.

Scanning

- Think posture all the time. Avoid bending, twisting, reaching, lifting, sustained pressure, arm abduction and awkward postures.
- Alternate sitting and standing and vary scanning techniques and transducer grip.
- Take time to adjust to all equipment and have accessories on hand before beginning the scan.
- Push rather than pull equipment.
- Get the patient to move as close as possible.
- Lower the couch to reduce arm abduction. This provides a more comfortable transducer grip and allows gravity to assist when applying pressure with the transducer.
- If the arm is abducted, support it by a cushion or rest it on the patient.
- Perform regular stretching, strengthening and aerobic exercises to maintain good fitness.
- Stretch before commencing work, in between examinations and at the end of the day.
- Rest and stretch the hand and wrist during procedures.
- Refocus eyes onto distant objects every few minutes.
- Discuss techniques with colleagues and exchange ideas to develop techniques that reduce stress on the body to avoid musculoskeletal injuries.

- Become multiskilled to vary work tasks.
- Follow infection control protocols at all times to prevent cross infection.
- Read literature and visit websites for workplace injuries, back care and specific musculoskeletal injuries in sonography.
- Report and document pain and discomfort then seek competent medical advice before undertaking any stretching, strengthening or aerobic exercise programme.

Workload and scheduling

- Organize appointments and introduce task rotation to avoid repetitive or successive similar ergonomically difficult examinations.
- Ensure adequate staffing levels to allow sonographers to take scheduled breaks to allow fatigued muscles to recover.
- Ensure that meal breaks are taken, to completely relax.

Patients

A signed referral specifying the area to be examined and clinical notes are required for each patient. If there is doubt, ring the referring doctor for clarification.

We provide patients with the following information:

- **What do you need to do before the test?** No preparation is required unless you are having an examination within the abdomen. If so, we provide instructions for fasting.
- **What does a test involve?** The test is completely non-invasive. There are no injections or other painful procedures. The energy levels for ultrasound are extremely low and there is no evidence that ultrasound, as used in these studies, can damage any structure within the body.
- **What will happen during the test?** A typical scan takes 30–60 min depending on the area being studied and how complex the scan is. There are no side-effects and you will be able to resume normal activities immediately. The room is darkened so that the sonographer can see the images better. You may be required to lie down, sit or stand, depending on the test. A non-staining

water-based gel is applied to the skin to provide contact for transmission of sound waves through the skin. Ultrasound is completely painless but pressure from the transducer may feel uncomfortable and you should report this to the sonographer.

For abdominal studies, we provide patients with the following instructions to avoid excessive gas. Preferably book these patients for morning scans as gas tends to accumulate during the day.

- **Nil orally**: diabetic patients should not fast. For all others:
    - for **24 hours** before the scan: avoid food and drink known to produce gas such as carbonated drinks, beer and dairy products
    - for **8 hours** before the scan: drink no more than small amounts of clear fluid. Cease smoking as this ingests air
    - for **1 hour** before a scan for the kidneys: drink several large glasses of water
    - take your medications as normal with a little food if required.

Patient safety

- **Cross-infection**: thoroughly clean and disinfect transducers before and after contact with any patient that might cause cross-infection. Use transducer sheaths if there is a prospect of contamination with blood or tissue discharges.
- **Injuries to the skin**: avoid damage to fragile skin by the transducer, your nails or jewellery.
- **Incident reports**: develop a procedure for a permanent record of untoward events or complications.

Sonographer's responsibilities

- Explain what is to be done.
- Ensure the patient has verbally consented.
- Ask if the scan is causing discomfort.
- Keep the patient informed as to how much longer the scan will take.
- Ask patients to move by themselves as much as possible.
- Be aware of patient privacy.
- Ensure the patient is adequately covered, especially when scanning in the groin.
- Seek permission to lean on a patient for arm support if required.

REPORTS

Preparing a report

- Use a checklist of headings and text for each test.
- A responsible physician must interpret and sign the report.
- Plan how information is to be conveyed to the referring physician.

The worksheet and final report must include:

- patient information
- date of scan
- indication for the examination
- study performed
- body of data (plaque, velocity, etc.)
- summary with final interpretation showing clinical relevance
- comparison with prior examinations
- sonographer name or initials
- physician signature.

Warning!

Indicate on the worksheet or report whether the examination was excellent, good or poor. Emphasize if a scan is suboptimal.

QUALITY ASSURANCE

Published criteria that define normal values and degrees of abnormality for duplex scans vary from centre to centre. Guidelines recommended in later chapters are a compromise and should not be blindly accepted as being absolutely correct. Whether published or internally generated criteria are used, they should always be internally validated by comparing results with other imaging techniques such as arteriography. Simple statistical techniques are required.

Observer variability

There is always a degree of variation for comparison of measurements for an individual sonographer made at different times (intraobserver variability) or between two sonographers (interobserver variability). It is not necessary to report values exactly and it is best to round velocities to the nearest 5 or 10 cm/s.

Variability can be calculated using Bland–Altman analysis (Fig. 3.1).

If a and b represent a pair of observations, then

$$\frac{(a + b)}{2} = \text{the mean of each pair}$$

This is plotted against

$$a - b = \text{the difference between each pair.}$$

The mean of the differences between all pairs of observations is

$$x = \frac{\sum (a + b)}{n}$$

(where n is the number of observations) and this should be close to zero.

The 95 per cent confidence limit for all observations is

$$\frac{2\sum (a - b)2}{(n - 1)}$$

Contingency tables

A particular value is chosen for each test to define a grade of disease. For example, it might be accepted that greater than 50 per cent diameter stenosis on an arteriogram or a peak systolic velocity >200 cm/s from a duplex scan each indicate that arterial disease that may require treatment is present.

Two-by-two contingency tables show how well these values detect disease. A new 'unknown' test is compared with an established

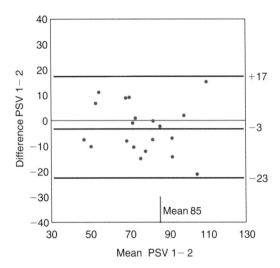

Fig. 3.1

Bland–Altman analysis: interobserver variability

Agreement between two sonographers for peak systolic velocities (PSV; cm/s) in the femoral artery. The mean of all measurements for both was 85 cm/s, the difference in means for all observations was 3 cm/s and 95 per cent confidence range was +17 to −23 cm/s. Observations would need to differ by >20 cm/s to represent a significant difference. Fig. 26.2 from Myers KA, Sumner DS and Nicolaides AN. 1997: *Lower Limb Ischaemia*. London: Medorion

standard of reference or 'gold standard' (Fig. 3.2). There is always an overlap in values for each so that the new test will apparently show many **true positive** (TP) and **true negative** (TN) results as well as a few **false positives** or 'false alarms' (FP) and **false negatives** or 'misses' (FN).

A highly sensitive test detects most patients with the abnormality so that a negative result for a sensitive test gives reassurance that all is well. A highly specific test identifies most normal subjects so that a positive result for a highly specific test gives confidence that disease is truly present.

$$\textbf{Accuracy} = \frac{(TP + TN)}{(TP + TN + FP + FN)}$$

– proportion of 'correct' tests to all tests performed.

$$\textbf{Positive predictive value} = \frac{(TP)}{(TP + FP)}$$

– likelihood that a subject with a positive test actually has the disease.

$$\textbf{Negative predictive value} = \frac{(TN)}{(TN + FN)}$$

– likelihood that a subject with a negative test does not have the disease.

$$\textbf{Sensitivity} = \frac{(TP)}{(TP + FN)}$$

– likelihood that a result will be positive if the subject actually has disease.

$$\textbf{Specificity} = \frac{(TN)}{(TN + FP)}$$

– likelihood that a result will be negative when the subject is truly free from disease.

$$\textbf{Positive likelihood ratio} = \frac{sensitivity}{(1 - specificity)}$$

– probability of a positive test in those with disease compared with the probability of a positive test in those without disease.

$$\textbf{Negative likelihood ratio} = \frac{(1 - sensitivity)}{(specificity)}$$

– probability of a negative test in those with disease compared with the probability of a negative test in those without disease.

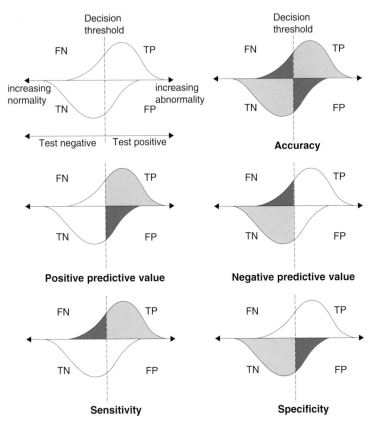

Fig. 3.2

Contingency tables

Pink areas represent true positive or negative results and red areas represent false positive or negative results. Fig. 26.4 from Myers KA, Sumner DS and Nicolaides AN. 1997: *Lower Limb Ischaemia*. London: Medorion.

Receiver operating characteristics (ROC) curves

Any value can be chosen to define abnormality. This can be selected using ROC curves (Fig. 3.3). Several values are chosen, and sensitivity and specificity are calculated for each and plotted against each other. The upper right section corresponds to high sensitivity and low specificity that indicates a 'lax threshold'. For example, it could mean

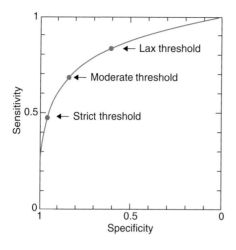

Fig. 3.3
ROC curve: prediction of failure after surgical intervention

that more patients with lower limb ischaemia would be considered for operation than is strictly necessary, which might be appropriate for patients with critical ischaemia. The lower left section corresponds to low sensitivity and high specificity for a 'strict threshold'. For example, it could mean that a patient with lower limb ischaemia who goes on to operation has really 'earned' the treatment and perhaps this is an appropriate bias for managing patients with claudication.

4

VASCULAR PHYSIOLOGY

Understanding pulsatile flow in compliant blood vessels is far more complex than applying physical laws relating to steady flow in rigid tubes, but the latter provide a guide. To date, clinical duplex scanning has been used to study larger blood vessels, and this chapter concentrates on these rather than the microcirculation.

BLOOD FLOW IN ARTERIES

Symbols used in the description and calculation of blood flow are shown in Box 4.1.

Box 4.1: Symbols used

- A: cross-sectional area (cm^2)
- d: diameter (cm)
- D: shear rate ($ml/s.cm^3$)
- g: acceleration due to gravity = $980\,cm/s^2$
- h: height (cm)
- l: length (cm)
- P: pressure (1 mmHg = 1333 dynes/cm^2)
- ΔP: pressure gradient between two sites
- Δp: pulse pressure at one site (systolic−diastolic pressure)
- Q: flow (ml/s)
- R: resistance
- r: internal radius (cm)
- Δr: change in radius with the pulse (mm)

- Re: Reynold's number for turbulence (dimensionless)
- t: arterial wall thickness (mm)
- v: velocity (cm/s)
- ρ: fluid density (gm/cm^3) = 1.056 for blood
- η: coefficient of viscosity (poise)
- T: shear stress (ml/s/cm^3)

Intravascular pressure, blood volume and flow velocity

The human circulation is a closed system of tubes containing blood under pressure. Blood flows in arteries due to propelling pressure (force per unit area) from left ventricular contraction. The volume flowing through an artery or sum of its branches averaged over time is constant. Flow velocity is proportional to cross-sectional area or radius such that:

$$Q = vA \text{ or } v = \frac{Q}{A} = \frac{Q}{\pi r^2}$$

Theoretically, if the diameter at an arterial stenosis is reduced by 50 per cent then the velocity should increase by four times but it is less than this in practice.

Energy for blood flow

Physical principles relating to flow in hollow tubes were initially studied assuming that fluid flows at a constant velocity, the tube is rigid, there is no energy loss along its length and fluid is incompressible. The driving pressure for flow within a tube is determined by its potential energy (PE) and kinetic energy (KE).

PE is the latent capacity to do work resulting from the fluid density, acceleration due to gravity, and height of the tube such that:

$$\text{PE} = \rho g h$$

PE results in considerable pressure variations in the human circulation in the standing position (Fig. 4.1).

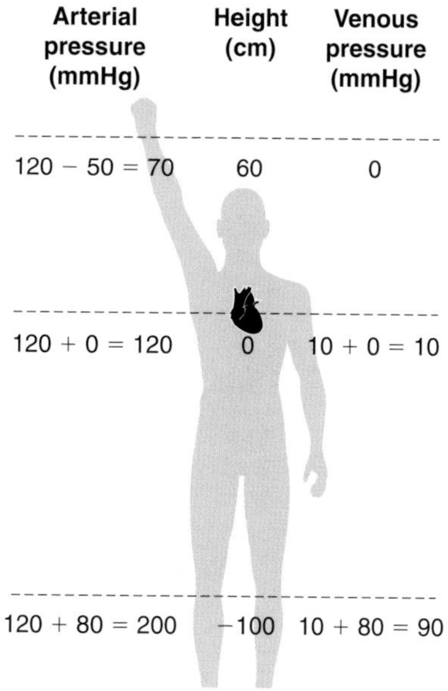

Arterial pressure (mmHg)	Height (cm)	Venous pressure (mmHg)
120 − 50 = 70	60	0
120 + 0 = 120	0	10 + 0 = 10
120 + 80 = 200	−100	10 + 80 = 90

Fig. 4.1

Potential energy

Fluid flows from a low pressure (high PE) at the heart or above to a high pressure (low PE) at the feet.

If $h = 100$ cm from heart to feet while standing, then:

$\Delta P = \rho g(h_2 - h_1)$
$= 1.056 \times 980 \times 100$
$= 103\,488$ dynes/cm^2
≈ 80 mmHg.

KE is the energy resulting from the fact that fluid is flowing. It is determined from fluid density and velocity such that:

$$KE = \frac{1}{2}\rho v^2$$

KE increases where a tube narrows (Fig. 4.2).

Conservation of energy requires that pressures at two points (1 and 2) along a tube are expressed as **Bernoulli's equation** (Daniel Bernoulli (1700–1782), a second generation member of a Swiss family of 12 eminent mathematicians):

$$P_1 + \rho g h_1 + \frac{1}{2}\rho v_1^2 = P_2 + \rho g h^2 + \frac{1}{2}\rho v_2^2, \text{ or:}$$
$$\Delta P + \rho g \left(h^2 - h_1\right) + \frac{1}{2}\rho \left(v_2^2 + v_1^2\right)$$

In some circumstances, v_1 is small compared with v_2 and the formula can be simplified to **Torricelli's equation** (Evangelista Torricelli

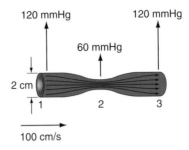

Fig. 4.2

Kinetic energy

Fluid flows from a low to high KE region at a narrowing to cause substantial pressure drop. If the inlet (1) has a diameter of 2 cm, fluid is flowing at 100 cm/s and the diameter at a narrowing (2) is 1 cm so that velocity theoretically increases to 400 cm/s, then

$$\Delta P = \frac{1}{2}\rho(v_2^2 - v_1^2)$$
$$= \frac{1}{2} \times 1.056(160\,000 - 10\,000)$$
$$= 79\,2000\ dynes/cm^2$$
$$\approx 60\ mmHg.$$

(1608–1647), an Italian physicist and mathematician):

$$\Delta P \approx \frac{1}{2}v_2^2$$

This is used to calculate stenoses in cardiac studies but the equations are not reliable for peripheral arterial studies.

Energy loss for arterial blood flow

These ideal circumstances for Bernoulli's equation do not apply to actual flow in arteries, in part because energy is lost from conversion to heat with persisting fall in pressure. This is due to the following factors.

Viscous drag in fluid and at the arterial wall

This represents a difference between 'ideal fluids' where all layers move at the same velocity and 'real fluids' where layers drag on each other. The concept is that there are infinite numbers of layers, each of which slides on the next like many cylinders (Fig. 4.3).

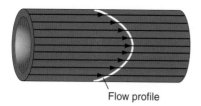

Fig. 4.3

Laminar flow

Steady flow of viscous fluid in a rigid tube with a circular cross-section produces a parabolic profile.

Flow profile

The theoretical fall in pressure due to viscosity causing loss of KE converted to heat is calculated from **Poiseuille's equation** (Jean-Louis-Marie Poiseuille (1799–1869), a French physician and physiologist):

$$\Delta P = \frac{8l\eta v}{\pi r^2} = \frac{8l\eta Q}{\pi r^4}$$

The coefficient of viscosity (η) is determined by 'shear stress' (T) which reflects the force required to slide one layer on another, and 'shear rate' (D) which is dependent on flow, such that

$$\eta = \frac{T}{D}$$
$$T = \frac{4\eta Q}{\pi r^3} \text{ and}$$
$$D = \frac{4Q}{\pi r^3}$$

The formulae show that pressure fall is much greater in vessels with a small radius in the microcirculation, and viscosity has minimal influence on flow in larger vessels. Blood viscosity decreases as flow velocity increases ('thixotropy'), but this is also only relevant in the microcirculation.

Disturbed flow

Fluid immediately adjacent to the wall is considered to be stationary, providing the concept of a thin 'boundary layer'. The boundary layer becomes thicker as flow becomes slower or if the wall is rough. It then tends to break up into small eddies or 'disturbed flow' (Fig. 4.4) and KE is lost by conversion to heat.

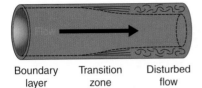

Fig. 4.4

Transition zone

Change at the wall from laminar boundary layer flow to disturbed flow.

Boundary layer   Transition zone   Disturbed flow

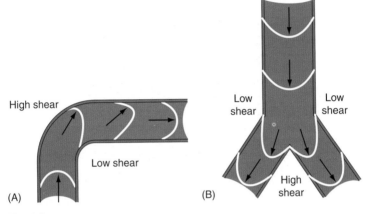

Fig. 4.5

Laminar flow at a curvature (A) or bifurcation (B)

The apex of the parabola moves away from the concave wall at a curve and outer wall at a bifurcation leading to areas of potential stagnation.

Blood flow in normal arteries is usually laminar but disturbed flow can develop with segments of stationary or reversed flow at sites of arterial dilatation, curvature, angulation, branching or bifurcation. Flow tends to be stable where flow is faster on the outside of a curve, and unstable where flow is slower on the inside of a curve (Fig. 4.5). Relatively stagnant flow may favour deposition of materials that lead to atherosclerosis or neo-intimal hyperplasia (see page 83 in Chapter 5).

'**Boundary layer separation**' is well recognized from Doppler ultrasound in the internal carotid artery (ICA) bulb (Fig. 4.6).

Similar disturbed flow at anastomoses between a bypass graft and artery can lead to areas of stagnant flow predisposing to recurrent disease causing stenosis (Fig. 4.7).

VASCULAR PHYSIOLOGY **65**

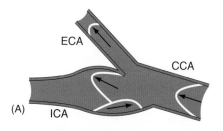

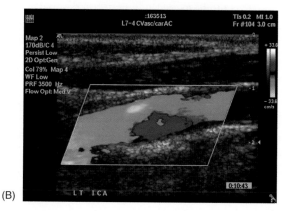

Fig. 4.6

Boundary layer separation

Reverse flow in the ICA bulb in a normal young patient. CCA: common carotid artery; ECA: external carotid artery.

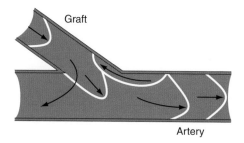

Fig. 4.7

Boundary layer separation

Reverse flow, vortices and stagnant flow at the angle of anastomosis for a bypass graft.

Turbulence

At a stage beyond disturbed flow, the pattern breaks up completely, resulting in chaotic fluid movements and very considerable energy loss and a fall in pressure that is not regained. Most energy is lost due to disturbed flow and turbulence at the entrance and exit of a stenosis.

The point at which flow breaks up is defined by **Reynold's number** – Re (Osborne Reynolds (1842–1912), a British engineer and physicist):

$$Re = \frac{vd\rho}{\eta}$$

Re is more likely to be exceeded in large arteries and at high velocities. Flow is commonly turbulent for Re > 2000. Reducing peripheral resistance by exercise or other stimuli causes an increased velocity across a stenosis which increases the likelihood of exceeding Re leading to turbulence and an even greater pressure fall.

Pressure changes at an arterial stenosis

KE loss at a stenosis causes a pressure drop dependent on the change in velocity between two points (1 and 2) such that

$$\Delta P = k(v_2 - v_1)^2 \text{ where } k \text{ is a constant.}$$

Blood flow through a stenosis starts to fall and peak systolic velocity rises when the diameter decreases to approximately 50 per cent and there is a sharp late fall in peak systolic velocity to 'trickle flow' beyond approximately 90–95 per cent stenosis (Fig. 4.8).

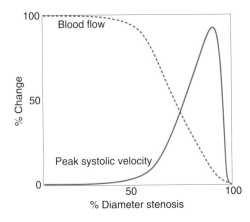

Fig. 4.8

Flow and velocity changes related to severity of arterial stenosis.

Flow becomes laminar again just beyond a stenosis but energy loss and fall in flow and pressure persist. This pressure drop is less than the fall calculated from Poiseuille's equation for viscosity alone. The value of the constant (k) depends more on the shape than the length of stenosis, with more flow disturbance if the stenosis is irregular or abrupt rather than smooth.

Measuring an arterial stenosis

Stenosis can be defined either by reduced diameter or cross-sectional area:

$$\text{Diameter of residual lumen} = \left(1 - \frac{r_2}{r_1}\right) \times 100\%$$

$$\text{Cross-sectional area of residual lumen} = \left(1 - \frac{r_2^2}{r_1^2}\right) \times 100\%$$

For example, if diameter is reduced by 50 per cent then area is reduced by 75 per cent.

There is a particular problem with defining ICA stenosis because two different techniques have been used to measure the normal ICA diameter (Fig. 4.9).

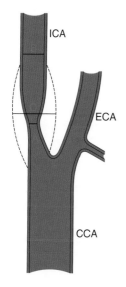

Fig. 4.9

Internal carotid artery stenosis

● Some reports define ICA stenosis from its diameter (A) relative to normal diameter distal to the stenosis (B) = ($B − A$)/B × 100 (ICA stenosis). We use this technique to grade stenosis by ultrasound.

● Other reports define ICA stenosis from its diameter (A) relative to that of the carotid bulb (C) at the level of stenosis = ($C − A$)/C × 100 (bulb stenosis).

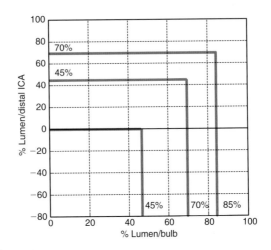

Fig. 4.10

Comparison of two methods for calculating ICA stenosis

- Bulb stenosis 45 per cent = ICA stenosis 0 per cent.
- Bulb stenosis 70 per cent = ICA stenosis 45 per cent.
- Bulb stenosis 85 per cent = ICA stenosis 70 per cent.

The bulb diameter is approximately 1.8 times distal ICA diameter. Calculations by the two methods results in considerable disparity (Fig. 4.10).

Pulsatile blood flow in arteries

Classical equations for flow are no more than an approximation to flow in arteries because blood flow is pulsatile and arteries are compliant and branching.

The arterial flow signal is a summation of forward flow from left ventricular contraction and reverse flow from tidal reflection shown in Fig. 4.11.

The profile for laminar flow changes throughout the pulse cycle is shown in Fig. 4.12.

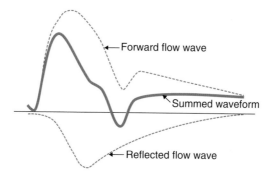

Fig. 4.11

Arterial pulse

Upper curve: left ventricular contraction causes forward flow with a systolic and diastolic component.

Lower curve: a water-hammer effect from flow striking major arterial branches as well as the peripheral resistance causes reverse flow.

Middle curve: the actual flow signal is a summation of the two.

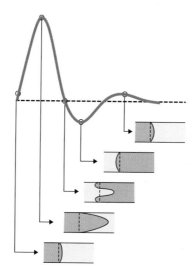

Fig. 4.12

Flow profile

The profile is flat at the start of the pulse when flow is minimal, becomes parabolic through systole, and then becomes mixed during diastole.

Resistance to flow

Turbulence and viscous drag cause resistance to flow:

$$R = \frac{\Delta P}{Q} = \frac{\Delta P}{v\pi r^2}$$

The smaller the diameter, the greater the resistance.

Resistances in parallel

As with electrical currents, resistance through each parallel pathway is greater than for the main channel alone:

$$\frac{1}{RT} = \frac{1}{R_1} + \frac{1}{R_2} + \cdots$$

Peripheral resistance

Resistance is much higher in smaller vessels so that the pressure drop mostly occurs in the microcirculation rather than larger branching arteries.

Spectral Doppler shows the resistance in an arterial bed (Fig. 4.13). Some sites such as the limbs and small intestine have an inherently **high-resistance circulation**. Pulse reflection results in low, absent or reversed flow in diastole. Other organs such as the brain or kidneys have an inherently **low-resistance circulation** with continuing forward flow through diastole.

Stimuli that induce vasodilatation in the microcirculation cause resistance to fall in high-resistance circulations. These include exercise in limb muscles, sympathetic blockade in skin, or food ingestion in the small intestine.

In many regions, resistance vessels in the microcirculation constrict if pressure rises and dilate if pressure falls, to maintain a relatively constant flow termed **autoregulation**.

Collateral resistance

Multiple collaterals that develop around an occluded artery have a total resistance in parallel that is far higher than resistance in

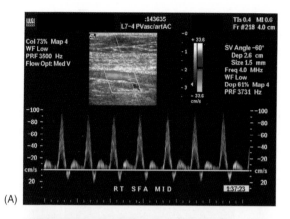

(A)

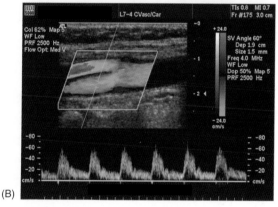

(B)

Fig. 4.13

Spectral tracings from an artery to:

A: a high-resistance circulation

B: a low-resistance circulation.

the normal native artery. The spectral Doppler signal through a collateral is high resistance. Collateral resistance around an arterial occlusion is less than peripheral resistance at rest even allowing pulses to be felt, but collateral resistance becomes greater if peripheral resistance is reduced by exercise so that the normal hyperaemic response is far less.

The spectral waveform proximal to a high-grade stenosis or occlusion is a high-resistance signal whereas the waveform distal to the lesion is 'dampened' and low resistance (Fig. 4.14).

Blood flow through an arterial bypass graft

The relative sizes of the graft and collateral bed determine how well the graft functions. At rest, resistance from either is so much less than the peripheral resistance that almost any graft will carry adequate flow, and it requires severe graft restenosis to cause a fall in pressure and flow.

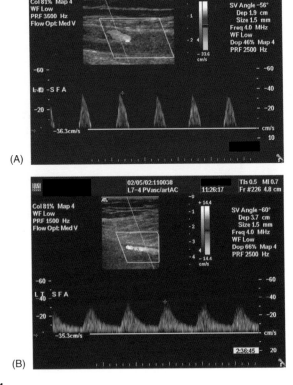

(A)

(B)

Fig. 4.14

Spectral tracing showing:

A: a high-resistance signal proximal to severe stenosis or occlusion

B: a dampened low-resistance signal distal to the lesion.

Resistances in series

As with electrical currents, resistance through each consecutive site is less than for the main channel alone:

$$RT = R_1 + R_2 + \cdots$$

Resistances for each stenosis combine to cause increased resistance to flow. Multiple short stenoses cause a larger fall in perfusion pressure and velocity than for one long stenosis alone.

Intermittent claudication

At rest, circulation to muscles is a high-resistance system. During exercise, muscle contraction releases vasodilator chemicals that cause arteriolar dilatation resulting in increased blood flow by some 10–20 times. Potential pain-producing metabolites are washed away and vasodilatation recedes within 30–60 s after stopping exertion. An arterial occlusion or severe stenosis increases resistance through collaterals so that peak increase in flow is much reduced and delayed (Fig. 4.15). Pain-producing metabolites accumulate above a pain threshold causing intermittent claudication (claudicare: to limp).

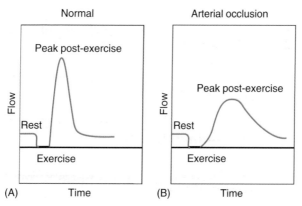

Fig. 4.15

Blood flow in the calf after a period of exercise:

A: in the normal circulation

B: in a limb with an arterial occlusion or severe stenosis.

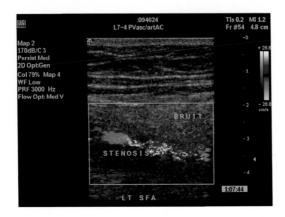

Fig. 4.16
Colour signals in tissues due to reverberations from the arterial wall at a site of turbulence corresponding to an arterial bruit.

Ischaemic rest pain

Unlike muscle, the skin circulation has very considerable sympathetic nervous control. Decreased perfusion pressure due to an arterial occlusion or severe stenosis is compensated by arteriolar dilatation until disease is advanced. There comes a stage where skin circulation is reduced beyond a point where compensation can occur, and metabolites accumulate that cause severe burning pain in the foot. This first becomes apparent at night due to decreased perfusion from the normal nocturnal fall in systemic blood pressure.

Arterial bruits

Turbulence in an artery causes its wall to vibrate and this produces a noise propagated through tissues that can be heard with a stethoscope or seen on an ultrasound scan (Fig. 4.16). It may require an increase in velocity by exercising to reduce peripheral resistance to cause sufficient turbulence to allow a bruit to be heard.

Changes in the wall of an aneurysm

Weakening in the wall allows it to progressively stretch and increase in diameter and length. Circumferential wall tension (T_c) in a cylindrical tube is

$$T_c = \frac{Pr}{t}$$

Wall tension increases as the radius increases and wall thickness decreases so as to allow more rapid expansion and eventual rupture.

BLOOD FLOW IN VEINS

Deep veins carry more than 80 per cent of the normal circulation. Two mechanisms cause blood to flow through veins to the heart:

- pressure transmitted through the microcirculation is small but constant. Venous flow is increased by vasodilatation with exercise and reduced by vasoconstriction caused by cold or arterial insufficiency
- pressure is exerted by intermittent contraction of adjacent muscles, particularly from the calf. During ultrasound examination, this is reproduced by squeezing relaxed calf muscles causing 'venous augmentation'.

Flow is modified by other influences:

- pulsatile contractions of the right atrium cause transient increases in venous pressure and arrest of flow which is restored as the atrium relaxes. This is only observed in central veins
- there are phasic variations of flow with respiration in proximal veins in the limbs although this is lost in distal veins
- changing intrathoracic pressures with respiration cause opposite effects in the upper and lower extremities. For veins in the upper extremities, inspiration results in an increase in pressure gradient to central veins, and venous flow increases. For veins in the lower extremity, inspiration causes the diaphragm to descend, increasing intra-abdominal pressure causing venous flow to slow, whereas lower limb venous flow increases during expiration
- increased intra-abdominal and intrathoracic pressure with straining or the Valsalva manoeuvre causes flow to slow or stop in all limbs.

Just as for branching arteries, resistance in each of the smaller veins in parallel is greater than resistance in a large vein such as the inferior vena cava. Accordingly, the larger the vein, the greater the flow velocity. Blood flow is most stagnant in smaller veins such as in the calf, making them more susceptible to venous thrombosis.

Reflux in lower limb veins from gravity, inspiration or straining is normally prevented by venous valves so that flow is only towards the heart. Valves become more numerous the further the vein is from the central circulation, and they are not present at all in the iliac veins or inferior vena cava.

5

VASCULAR PATHOLOGY

Arterial disease is most commonly caused by atherosclerosis but there are several uncommon or rare non-atherosclerotic arterial diseases. Aneurysmal arterial disease may have a pathogenesis different from atherosclerosis. The causes of chronic venous disease are not fully understood but there is disturbance of normal venous flow due to valvular incompetence or venous obstruction. Thrombosis can complicate any arterial or venous disease. This chapter describes diseases that may be manifest at various sites, and conditions specific to a particular site are discussed in regional chapters.

NORMAL ARTERIAL STRUCTURE AND FUNCTION

The wall of a large artery has three layers (Fig. 5.1):

● the **intima** is a single layer of endothelial cells supported by a continuous basement membrane and internal elastic lamina. Endothelial cells:
  ● regulate haemostasis and thrombosis
  ● interact with white blood cells
  ● produce growth factors
  ● are permeable to nutrients
  ● control vascular tone
● the **media** contains smooth muscle cells (SMCs) responsible for:
  ● muscle contraction to maintain vascular tone, or
  ● synthesizing a matrix of collagen, elastin and glycoproteins

● The **adventitia** consists of fibroblasts in a matrix of collagen and glycoproteins.

Ultrasound can distinguish the three layers and measure intima–media thickness (Fig. 5.2) which relates well to future risk for clinical arterial disease.

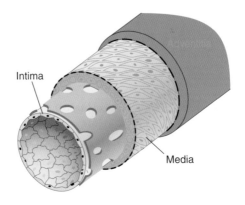

Fig. 5.1

Three layers of an arterial wall

Fig. 12.2a from Myers KA, Marshall RD and Freidin J. 1980: *Principles of Pathology*. Oxford: Blackwell. Reproduced with permission from Blackwell.

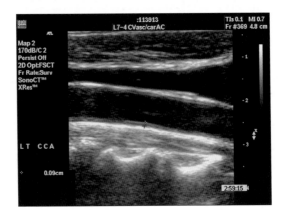

Fig. 5.2

B-mode of layers of a normal arterial wall showing intima–media thickness, best measured on the far wall.

HAEMOSTASIS AND THROMBOSIS

Normal haemostasis is balanced to prevent excessive bleeding after a vascular injury while preventing spontaneous intravascular clotting. There are three major factors responsible for controlling haemostasis:

- **endothelial cells** in the wall oppose clotting since they prevent platelets from adhering to subendothelial structures, possess anticoagulant properties from heparin-like molecules, and contain fibrinolytic factors that clear fibrin deposits on the wall
- **platelets** adhere to subendothelial collagen after endothelial disruption. This sets off a series of reactions known as platelet activation resulting in platelet aggregation to form a platelet plug. Damaged endothelial cells release von Willebrand's factor essential for platelet adhesion to collagen
- **the coagulation system** results from a series of reactions that lead to conversion of fibrinogen to fibrin. Fibrin combines with platelet aggregates to cement the platelet plug. Damaged endothelial cells release factors that activate clotting pathways and depress fibrinolysis. The coagulation system is balanced by a number of anticoagulant factors that restrict clotting to the site of endothelial injury.

Thrombosis from haematological abnormalities

Arterial or venous thrombosis can result from:

- **hyperviscosity** due to haematological diseases that increase levels of red cells, white cells or serum proteins such as polycythaemia, lymphomas and leukaemias, or globulin disorders
- **thrombophilia** associated with congenital or acquired clotting factor abnormalities with:
  - deficiencies of normal clotting factors such as antithrombin III, protein C or protein S, or
  - the presence of abnormal clotting factors such as Leidin Factor V, antiphospholipid antibodies or homocysteine.

Venous thrombosis

Venous thrombosis results from three different processes referred to as Virchow's triad (Rudolf Ludwig Karl Virchow (1821–1902), a

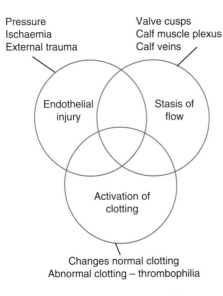

Pressure
Ischaemia
External trauma

Valve cusps
Calf muscle plexus
Calf veins

Endothelial injury

Stasis of flow

Activation of clotting

Changes normal clotting
Abnormal clotting – thrombophilia

Fig. 5.3

Virchow's triad

Three factors interact to predispose to venous thrombosis:

● stasis of blood flow
● endothelial injury
● activation of clotting.

German pathologist) (Fig. 5.3). Deep vein thrombosis (DVT) in the lower limbs with a risk of pulmonary embolism (PE) are particularly important (see Chapter 9).

Major risk factors that predispose to venous thromboembolism are:

● immobility
● trauma
● sepsis
● pregnancy
● obesity
● older age
● malignancy
● varicose veins
● previous DVT.

DVT or PE most often occur in the following settings:

● **surgery**. They are frequent, particularly after lower limb orthopaedic operations. Factors during operation that increase risk include poor hydration, immobility, a prolonged operation and deep anaesthesia

- **intravenous lines and catheters.** Devices used to infuse nutrients or drugs are often required for long periods, and are subject to a risk of causing thrombosis, particularly in the upper limbs (see page 317 in Chapter 16)
- **pregnancy.** DVT occurs in less than 1 in 1000 pregnancies but PE is a leading cause of maternal mortality. DVT is more common after Caesarean section and with advanced maternal age or obesity
- **oral contraceptives and hormone replacement therapy.** Both low-dose oestrogen oral contraceptives and progestagens for hormone replacement therapy increase the risk
- **medical diseases.** Myocardial infarction, heart failure, stroke, respiratory disease or cancer lead to a high risk of DVT that is increased by age or chemotherapy
- **thrombophilia.** Approximately 25 per cent of patients with idiopathic DVT have thrombophilia. Thrombosis due to thrombophilia often only occurs under other high-risk conditions
- **travel-related thrombosis.** There is an increased risk for DVT with prolonged air travel, and approximately two-thirds have associated medical disorders, hormone prescription or thrombophilia.

Pathogenesis

DVT is considerably more common in lower than upper limbs.

- **Propagation.** Thrombosis commonly commences in calf veins, particularly at valve sinuses. Thrombus can propagate along a vein, initially 'free floating' and not fixed to the wall, subsequently becoming adherent.
- **Recanalization.** With time, the vein wall produces thrombolytic factors that can recanalize the vein. However, this usually causes irreversible damage to venous valves so that venous reflux then occurs under the effect of gravity. Some 75 per cent of DVTs recanalize within 6 months and approximately two-thirds of these develop deep venous reflux.
- **Occlusion.** If inherent thrombolysis is ineffective then there will be persisting occlusion. Whether or not veins remain permanently occluded or reopen is unpredictable and depends in part on the extent of thrombosis and efficacy of treatment. The lumen is filled

with thrombus for up to several months. Later, the vein may remain filled with a mucoid material but more often becomes completely sclerosed as a fibrous cord. Collateral veins develop to a varying degree.

ATHEROSCLEROSIS

Aetiology

This complex process involves blood contents, endothelial cells and SMCs in the media (Fig. 5.4).

Risk factors

There is an inherent risk of atherosclerosis to varying degrees in all people. Arterial injury and lipid accumulation is accentuated by risk factors including:

- smoking
- diabetes mellitus

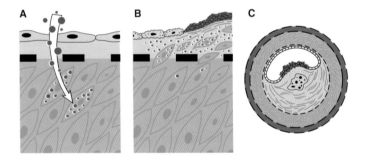

Fig. 5.4

Initiation of atherosclerosis

A: Endothelial damage by chemical or mechanical injuries activates white blood cells, platelets and endothelial cells to produce chemical factors that cause changes in the underlying media.

B: SMCs react by migrating from the media into the subendothelial plane.

C: SMCs proliferate and change from contractile cells to synthesizing lipid-rich foam cells; secondary degeneration releases lipid, and platelets aggregate on the surface.

Fig. 12.5 from Myers KA, Marshall RD and Freidin J. 1980: *Principles of Pathology*. Oxford: Blackwell. Reproduced with permission from Blackwell.

- hypertension
- hyperlipidaemia
- homocystinaemia.

Pathology

Lesions tend to be patchy and concentrated at common sites. Disease is more likely to occur where flow is relatively stagnant against the arterial wall such as the aortic bifurcation (Fig. 5.5) allowing more prolonged contact of injurious agents with the wall (see page 64 in Chapter 4).

There is a progression of lesions:

- **the fatty streak** is the early phase with subendothelial aggregation of lipid-rich foam cells. It occurs from childhood but does not correspond to later distribution of clinical atherosclerosis
- **fibrous plaque** is a more advanced lesion with aggregates of subendothelial SMCs surrounded by connective tissue and lipid covered by a fibrous cap consisting of SMCs and connective tissue
- **an atheroma** contains lipid that accumulates as foam cells break down. Vasa vasora in the base of the plaque may haemorrhage

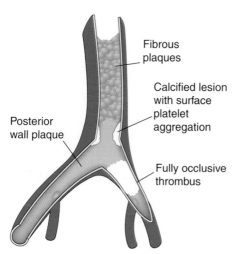

Fibrous plaques

Calcified lesion with surface platelet aggregation

Posterior wall plaque

Fully occlusive thrombus

Fig. 5.5

Changes due to atherosclerosis at the aortic bifurcation

Fig. 12.2f from Myers KA, Marshall RD and Freidin J. 1980: *Principles of Pathology*. Oxford: Blackwell. Reproduced with permission from Blackwell.

into its core increasing its size. Eventually, the swollen plaque may rupture, discharging embolic contents into the lumen and leaving a surface ulcer. Platelets aggregate to form another potential source of emboli

- **calcified plaque** results from secondary degeneration causing an inflammatory response with repair leading to a mixed lesion of fibrous tissue, lipid and increasing amounts of secondary calcification. The surface is irregular and this may cause thrombus and platelets to aggregate and embolize. However, there is less lipid in the plaque and a reduced risk of discharge of contents

- **arterial thrombosis** may be precipitated by rupture of the plaque, releasing substances that promote coagulation. Alternatively, progressive plaque degeneration can cause the arterial lumen to progressively narrow and eventually occlude. Unlike veins, there is no inherent mechanism for spontaneous thrombolysis, and recanalization of occluded arteries is rare.

Varying amounts of lipid, fibrous tissue and calcification in a plaque result in a range of pathological changes. These are reflected by B-mode ultrasound appearances (Fig. 5.6).

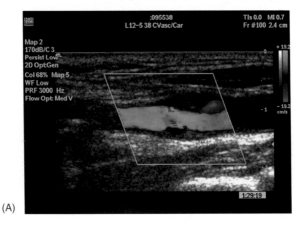

(A)

Fig. 5.6

B-mode appearances of atheromatous plaques

A: A lipid-rich plaque resulting in a homogeneous echolucent appearance only apparent as a filling defect with colour Doppler.

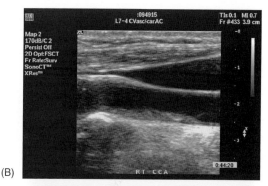

(B)

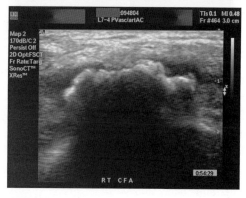

(C)

(D)

Fig. 5.6 (*continued*)

B: A diffusely fibrous plaque resulting in a homogeneous echogenic appearance.

C: A plaque containing various combinations of lipid, fibrous tissue and calcification resulting in a heterogeneous plaque.

D: 'Cauliflower' calcification causing acoustic shadowing.

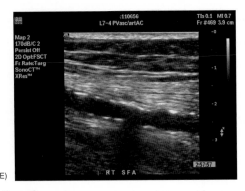

(E)

Fig. 5.6 (*continued*)

E: Diffuse calcification causing plaques along a considerable length of artery.

Pathogenesis

- Disease must narrow an artery to a 'critical stenosis' before significant symptoms develop.
- Acute thrombosis can supervene on minor stenosis producing acute ischaemia as the first presentation.
- Chronic occlusion may follow from critical stenosis. Occlusion extends between major branches that connect to form collateral arteries around the occlusion. The severity of symptoms depends in part on how well collaterals form.
- Small particles from an atheroma or secondary surface thrombus can detach to cause patchy infarcts from an embolism.

ARTERIAL ANEURYSMS

Aetiology

Degenerative aneurysms can affect any major artery from the aortic arch to distal major branches. Factors that predispose include:

- **heredity**: family clusters occur and first-degree male relatives are four times more likely to have an aneurysm
- **deficiencies of genetically linked enzymes** responsible for collagen cross-linking
- **impaired blood supply** from an intraluminal thrombus acting as a barrier to oxygen diffusion to the arterial wall, causing hypoxic necrosis

● **atherosclerotic plaques** that atrophy leaving a thin weak wall.

Other types of aneurysm include:

● **aneurysms associated with inflammatory arteritis**
● **mycotic aneurysms** from infection in the artery wall.

Risk factors

● Family history
● Hypertension
● Smoking
● Chronic obstructive pulmonary disease
● Atherosclerotic arterial disease elsewhere

Pathology

There are various configurations (Fig. 5.7):

Fusiform and saccular aneurysms

Both collagen and elastin degenerate in the wall and calcium is deposited. Atherosclerotic lesions make the remaining wall weak and

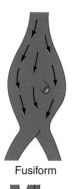

Fusiform

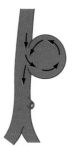

Saccular

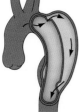

Dissecting

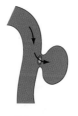

False

Fig. 5.7

Types of aneurysm

● **Fusiform:** involving the entire circumference of the aortic wall.
● **Saccular:** involving just a portion of the aortic circumference.
● **Dissecting:** with a false lumen.
● **False:** from arterial trauma.

From Fig. 13.10 from Queral L, in: Bergan JJ and Yao JS. 1979: *Surgery of the Aorta and its Body Branches*. New York: Grune and Stratton. Reproduced with permission.

brittle. Tangential stress from intravascular pressure is greater at certain sites, predisposing to local dilatation. Laminated thrombus accumulates on the degenerate inner arterial wall. Elastic retraction is lost, the diameter progressively increases and the aneurysmal artery gradually becomes more elongated and tortuous.

Dissecting aneurysm

Aortic dissection can commence with a tear in the intima from the start of the aortic arch, from just beyond the left subclavian artery, or less frequently from within the abdominal aorta or internal carotid artery (Fig. 6.13, page 112). It is caused by necrosis in the media and is common in diseases with congenital weakness from collagen deficiency from **Marfan's syndrome** or **Ehlers–Danlos syndrome**. Presentation may be acute with occlusion of aortic branches or iliac arteries, or the process may be chronic with aortic aneurysm formation.

False aneurysm

Arterial trauma, either accidental or iatrogenic, can cause a defect in the artery wall. Haemorrhage leads to a local haematoma and the breach in the artery frequently seals. However, arterial pressure can keep the opening patent so that pulsating blood progressively forms an aneurysmal space outside the lumen, compressing the haematoma into the wall.

NON-ATHEROSCLEROTIC ARTERIAL DISEASES

Several uncommon non-atherosclerotic arterial diseases should be considered, particularly in younger patients who lack major risk factors for atherosclerosis.

Inflammatory arterial diseases

There are several diseases with similar pathology but different clinical presentations that are probably caused by an immune reaction. They may be distinguished by ultrasound, but many have characteristic arteriographic findings and some even require arterial biopsy for diagnosis.

Takayasu's (pulseless) disease is common in Asia and affects children and young adults with a marked female preponderance (Mikita Takayasu (1860–1938), a Japanese ophthalmologist). Inflammation affects all layers of the aorta and its major branches to the cerebrovascular or visceral circulations, or to the extremities. An acute inflammatory phase with non-specific 'rheumatic-like' illness is followed years later by a chronic fibrotic phase that leads to large artery stenoses or occlusion, and aneurysms in some 30 per cent of cases. Homogeneous circumferential intima–media thickening is a highly specific finding on ultrasound.

Buerger's disease (thromboangiitis obliterans) usually occurs in young males, particularly from southern and eastern Europe, Israel or Asia, and always in smokers (Leo Buerger (1879–1943), an American surgeon). An early acute phase with inflammation in the arterial and venous wall and surrounding tissues causing thrombotic occlusion is followed by a chronic phase with fibrosis and collateral formation. Approximately 60 per cent have lower limb symptoms, 30 per cent have upper limb symptoms and 10 per cent have both, but arteriography shows changes in most arteries of all limbs indicating that disease is more extensive than predicted from symptoms.

Temporal (giant cell) arteritis predominantly affects women, is found in most countries, and is almost exclusively confined to the white population. The disease particularly affects temporal arteries but can occur in arteries to the extremities.

Behçet's syndrome is most prevalent in young males from eastern Mediterranean countries or Japan (Hulusi Behçet (1889–1948), a Turkish dermatologist). The pathology is non-specific inflammation in small and large vessels. Major arterial or venous thrombosis can occur at any site. Aneurysms particularly affect large arteries or sites of surgical anastomosis or arterial puncture, and they are frequently multiple.

Scleroderma is adventitial fibrosis that usually affects small arteries in the hands leading to Raynaud's phenomenon (see page 233 in Chapter 11) but it can also cause occlusion of large arteries to the limbs as a result of intimal hyperplasia.

Intrinsic diseases of the arterial wall

Aortic coarctation is a congenital segment of aortic hypoplasia, often with associated visceral and renal artery stenosis. It occurs in the thoracic aorta and occasionally high in the abdominal aorta. It should be considered in young patients with hypertension from decreased renal perfusion, an aortic bruit and lower limb ischaemia.

Fibromuscular dysplasia usually involves one or both renal arteries, but can affect other visceral arteries, extracranial internal carotid arteries (Fig. 6.11, page 111) or external iliac arteries. Most patients are female and aged less than 60 years. There is a series of stenoses with intervening dilatations.

Arterial trauma

Acute arterial trauma is a common indication for ultrasound assessment. Penetration through the arterial wall leads to major haemorrhage. However, many injuries rupture the intima and media leaving an intact adventitia. This can cause arterial occlusion and ischaemia. In very large arteries, the lumen may remain patent and the weakened wall becomes aneurysmal, either early or delayed.

Repetitive arterial trauma can cause subintimal fibrosis with stenosis, degeneration with aneurysm formation or thrombotic occlusion and is described in regional chapters.

Iatrogenic trauma can result from several procedures such as:

● arterial catheterization for arteriography
● intra-arterial infusions of therapeutic agents
● thrombosed arterial reconstructions.

Post-irradiation arteritis can cause endothelial damage in major arteries, usually manifest more than one to two years after radiation treatment. Consequent fibrosis extends through the wall, leading to arterial stenosis or occlusion.

Ergotism from oral administration of ergot preparations for migraine results from arterial spasm of large arteries to the limbs or aortic arch branches. Spasm in the early stages is completely reversible within a few hours of stopping the drug but endothelial damage can lead to thrombosis.

CHRONIC VENOUS DISEASE

Chronic venous disease predominantly affects the lower extremities. It is necessary to describe the normal lower limb venous circulation to be able to understand haemodynamic changes from superficial or deep venous reflux that lead to varicose veins and other changes.

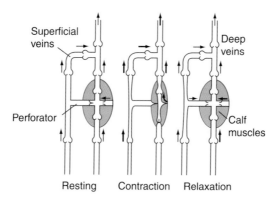

Fig. 5.8

Flow with muscle contraction in the normal venous circulation

- Resting: blood flows so that valves are open and pressure in the vein is the hydrostatic pressure from the heart.
- Contraction: blood is expelled from deep veins towards the heart.
- Relaxation: valves close and blood cannot reflux into deep or superficial veins; pressure in deep veins falls, pressure is higher in superficial veins, and blood flows from superficial to deep veins through the saphenous junctions and perforators.
- Blood enters through the microcirculation but usually with insufficient time to refill deep veins before the next muscle contraction so that ambulatory venous pressure remains well below the hydrostatic pressure.

Fig. 129-17 from Sumner DS. In: Rutherford RB. 1995: *Vascular Surgery*. Philadelphia: WB Saunders. Reproduced with permission.

Normal flow in lower limb veins

Valves in deep and superficial veins allow flow to pass to the heart and prevent blood from refluxing back to the periphery under the effect of gravity. Deep and superficial veins are connected by perforating veins at various levels in the lower limbs and these normally have valves that direct flow from superficial to deep veins.

Venous return has a small driving force through the capillary bed but largely depends on calf and thigh muscle pumping (Fig. 5.8).

Superficial venous reflux

Valves may be congenitally absent, may fail to coapt due to venous dilatation, or may be destroyed by recanalization after thrombosis.

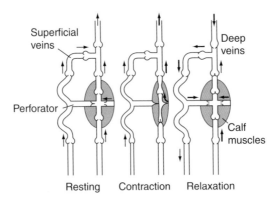

Fig. 5.9

Flow with muscle contraction in limbs with superficial venous reflux and varicose veins

- Resting: blood flows so that valves are open and pressure in a vein is the hydrostatic pressure from the heart.
- Contraction: blood is expelled from deep veins towards the heart and out to the surface through incompetent perforators.
- Relaxation: blood flows retrogradely through incompetent connections into superficial veins and varices, and a pressure gradient causes blood to flow inwards through perforators from distended superficial veins to emptied deep veins.
- Deep veins fill at a greater rate, and ambulatory venous pressure in deep and superficial veins is higher than normal.

Fig. 129-12 from Sumner DS. In: Rutherford RB. 1995: *Vascular Surgery*. Philadelphia: WB Saunders. Reproduced with permission.

Reflux will then occur due to gravity. Blood can flow through deep to superficial connections at the saphenous junctions, perforators or other sites (Fig. 5.9).

The resultant increased pressure leads to progressive dilatation and degeneration to form varicose veins (see Chapter 10). Varicose veins are twice as frequent in women compared with men, and other **risk factors** are obesity and multiparity. Patients may inherit weak vein walls or absent valves but a family history may simply reflect that the condition is common.

The evidence is that normal hydrostatic pressures distend abnormally weak veins and that the process does not result from abnormally high pressures distending normal veins. This is a generalized process and controlling one diseased segment is not likely to lead to permanent cure at all sites.

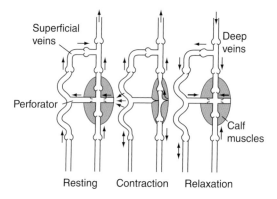

Fig. 5.10

Flow with muscle contraction in limbs with deep venous reflux

- Resting: blood flows so that valves are open and pressure in the veins is the hydrostatic pressure from the heart.
- Contraction: blood is expelled from deep veins towards the heart and out through perforators to superficial veins under high pressure.
- Relaxation: blood immediately flows backwards past incompetent valves, there is no pressure gradient between distended superficial veins and deep veins, and blood pools in both.
- Deep veins fill immediately and ambulatory venous pressure in deep and superficial veins is equal to the hydrostatic pressure.

Fig. 129-20 from Sumner DS. In: Rutherford RB. 1995: *Vascular Surgery*. Philadelphia: WB Saunders. Reproduced with permission.

Deep venous reflux

Valves in deep veins may be congenitally absent, present but not functioning, or destroyed by past DVT with recanalization. This leads to more severe venous hypertension (Fig. 5.10).

Perforator incompetence

There is speculation as to how varicose veins evolve. One school considers that primary incompetence at either saphenous junction causes progressive retrograde distension. If so, then perforators may be an important pathway to allow blood to escape from superficial varices into deep veins, and they should be preserved when treating venous disease. An opposing school considers that the primary source is from outflow through perforators causing antegrade distension. If so, they should be interrupted as part of treatment for varicose veins. Both are observed with ultrasound in early disease but the former is more common. Either mechanism may be present in different patients, but there is no definitive way to distinguish whether perforators are draining or feeding superficial veins.

Venous obstruction

Thrombus in a deep vein may fail to recanalize leading to long-term chronic obstruction. Pressures in deep veins increase with calf muscle contraction, forcing blood to pass out through perforators leading to severe superficial venous hypertension. Saphenous veins and their major tributaries are collaterals for outflow and cannot be removed for fear of further restricting outflow and worsening symptoms.

Proximal iliocaval obstruction can be inferred from the waveform in the common femoral vein with spectral analysis. Normal phasic variations with respiration and the response to the Valsalva manoeuvre are altered (Fig. 5.11).

Post-thrombotic syndrome

This term has long been used to describe chronic venous disease associated with complications due to damage to skin and fat in

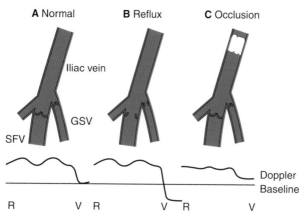

Fig. 5.11

Flow patterns with spectral analysis in the common femoral vein

R: respiratory fluctuations; V: Valsalva manoeuvre; SFV: superficial femoral vein; GSV: great saphenous vein.

A: Normal circulation; R: normal; V: causes flow to stop.

B: Superficial or deep reflux; R: normal; V: reverse flow.

C: Proximal obstruction; R: heavily dampened or lost; V: reduced or lost.

the leg. It was previously thought that complications were always associated with deep venous reflux or obstruction due to past DVT causing perforator incompetence. However, duplex scanning has shown that the larger proportion of complications result from superficial reflux alone.

6

EXTRACRANIAL CEREBROVASCULAR DISEASE

Duplex scanning identifies the presence, severity and type of disease in extracranial arteries. Stroke is the third most common cause of death in western countries and about 75 per cent of cases are due to thromboembolism from carotid arteries. Ultrasound is now used by many clinicians as the sole investigation to determine the best treatment for cerebrovascular disease.

ANATOMY

Box 6.1: Arteries scanned for reporting

- Common carotid artery: CCA
- Internal carotid artery: ICA
- External carotid artery: ECA
- Vertebral artery
- Innominate (brachiocephalic) artery
- Subclavian artery

Ultrasound can study aortic arch branches (Fig. 6.1), extracranial carotid arteries (Fig. 6.2) and vertebral arteries (Fig. 6.3, page 100).

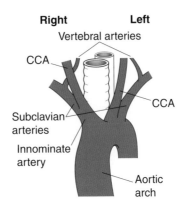

Fig. 6.1

Aortic arch branches

● Innominate artery divides into right subclavian artery and right CCA.
● Left subclavian artery and left CCA originate directly from the aortic arch.
● Variations occur: left CCA arises from innominate artery in 20–35 per cent.

Redrawn from Lord RSA. 1986: *Surgery of Occlusive Cerebrovascular Disease*. St Louis: CV Mosby. By kind permission of the author.

CLINICAL ASPECTS

Regional pathology

Disease can reduce perfusion pressure and flow. This is compensated by collaterals and intracranial vasodilatation termed **autoregulation**. Blood flow is not restricted until the lumen diameter is reduced by >50 per cent.

Sites of disease

Carotid and arch branch disease can be combined, as can extracranial and intracranial disease (Fig. 6.4).

Osteophytes can compress a vertebral artery in the cervical canal, often induced by turning the head. Thromboembolism can result from vertebral artery disease at any level.

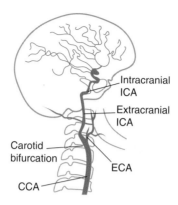

Fig. 6.2

Carotid arteries

- Lie deep to the sternomastoid muscle.
- The CCA is medial to the internal jugular vein and vagus nerve.
- The carotid bifurcation is usually at the angle of the mandible.
- The ECA is anteromedial to the ICA at the bifurcation.
- The ICA is larger than the ECA.
- The ICA and CCA usually have no extracranial branches.
- The ECA has multiple branches: the first is the superior thyroid artery.

Fig. 12.1c from Myers KA, Marshall RD and Freidin J. 1980: *Principles of Pathology*. Oxford: Blackwell. Reproduced with permission from Blackwell.

Subclavian or innominate steal syndrome

Subclavian or innominate artery disease can cause reversed ipsilateral vertebral artery flow to provide collateral circulation to 'steal' blood flow from the brain to the upper extremity (Fig. 6.5). The left subclavian artery is most commonly affected.

Non-atherosclerotic diseases

There are other uncommon or rare diseases.

- **Fibromuscular dysplasia** usually involves the mid to distal extracranial ICA on both sides.
- **Carotid artery dissection** commences with a flap of intima and media from the ICA origin through the length of ICA, although it can start in the CCA or arch.

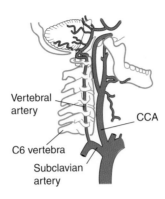

Fig. 6.3

Vertebral arteries

- Usually arise from the proximal subclavian arteries.
- Often differ in calibre.
- Lie lateral and posterior to the carotid arteries.
- Pass to a canal in the cervical vertebrae, usually entering at C6.
- Enter the skull through the foramen magnum.
- Join to form the basilar artery.

Fig. 10.2 from Moore WS. 1980: *Surgery for Cerebrovascular Disease.* Philadelphia: WB Saunders. Reproduced with permission.

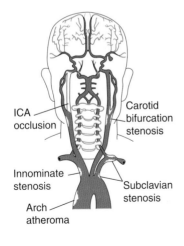

Fig. 6.4

Common sites for extracranial arterial disease

The most common site is at the carotid bifurcation with plaque extending into the ICA, usually with a discrete end-point.

Redrawn from Lord RSA. 1986: *Surgery of Occlusive Cerebrovascular Disease.* St Louis: CV Mosby. By kind permission of the author.

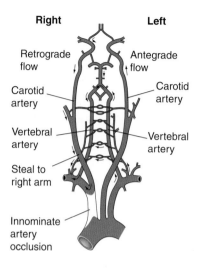

Right **Left**

Retrograde flow

Antegrade flow

Carotid artery

Carotid artery

Vertebral artery

Vertebral artery

Steal to right arm

Innominate artery occlusion

Fig. 6.5

'Steal' from brain to right arm from innominate artery occlusion

● Antegrade flow in the left vertebral and retrograde flow in the right vertebral artery.
● Reverse flow in the basilar artery.
● Flow through the circle of Willis to the basilar artery.
● Reverse flow in the right ICA and CCA.

Redrawn from Lord RSA. 1986: *Surgery of Occlusive Cerebrovascular Disease*. St Louis: CV Mosby. By kind permission of the author.

● **Carotid aneurysm** usually involves the distal CCA and proximal ICA and arterial dilatation is associated with mural thrombus.
● **Carotid body tumour** is a highly vascular 'paraganglionoma' usually seen in the bifurcation between the ICA and ECA but sometimes higher to the base of skull.
● **Takayasu's ('pulseless') disease** usually causes occlusion or aneurysms of major arch branches although it can extend to more distal arteries.
● **Temporal (giant cell) arteritis** affects the superficial temporal arteries in older women.

● Moya-Moya syndrome ('puffs of smoke') affects children to cause multiple occlusions or high-grade stenoses of extracranial carotid and vertebral arteries.

Clinical presentations

Disease can be asymptomatic. A cervical bruit can result from stenosis or tortuosity. Transient or persisting symptoms with neurological deficit can be due to embolism or flow restriction due to stenosis or occlusion.

Symptomatic carotid territory disease

ICA or CCA disease can cause:

● transient ischaemic attacks (TIAs): contralateral motor or sensory disturbance or speech impairment, defined as lasting less than 24 hours
● amaurosis fugax: transient ipsilateral monocular complete or partial loss of vision
● stroke or blindness.

Vertebrobasilar insufficiency

Vertebral or basilar artery disease, extrinsic vertebral artery compression in the spinal canal or subclavian or innominate steal syndrome can cause:

● visual disturbances and diplopia
● vertigo
● parasthesiae
● impaired coordination
● drop attacks.

Extrinsic vertebral artery compression usually causes transient, stereotyped symptoms. Thromboembolic ischaemia usually causes persistent, varied symptoms independent of head movements, and is at risk of causing stroke.

Differential diagnosis

● Cerebral embolism from cardiac mural thrombus due to atherosclerotic heart disease or atrial myxoma.

- Cerebral embolism from thrombus or vegetations on heart valves due to atrial fibrillation, rheumatic heart disease, subacute bacterial endocarditis or mitral valve prolapse.
- Vasospasm of intracranial arteries from migraine or subarachnoid haemorrhage.
- Postural hypotension.
- Transient hypoglycemia.
- Inner ear disease such as Ménière's syndrome or middle ear infection causing dizziness, vertigo, tinnitus and loss of balance.

Treatment

Lesser degrees of disease are best treated by medical measures. More severe stenosis is conventionally treated by carotid endarterectomy (CEA) or more recently by carotid stenting. Randomized trials show that CEA is superior to medical treatment for patients with >60–70 per cent stenosis, but every surgeon has a personal opinion as to the degree of stenosis that warrants CEA.

Warning!

It can be difficult to distinguish tight stenosis from occlusion. A completely occluded ICA cannot be corrected by surgery and will not release emboli. However, very severe stenosis can be a potential source for emboli or acute thrombosis and may require urgent surgery.

What the doctors need to know

- Is disease present?
- Which arteries are affected by disease and are they stenosed or occluded?
- What is the degree of carotid stenosis and nature of carotid plaques?
- Where is the carotid bifurcation and are there features that could make CEA more difficult – high bifurcation, tortuosity, coils and kinks, plaque extension or a narrow artery?

● What is the flow direction in vertebral arteries and are they normal, stenosed, occluded or absent?
● Can aortic arch branches be seen and are they normal or diseased?
● Is the scan quality adequate to allow reliable management decisions without the need for arteriography?

THE DUPLEX SCAN

Box 6.2: Abbreviations
● PSV: peak systolic velocity
● EDV: end diastolic velocity
● PSB: pansystolic spectral broadening

Normal findings

● The ICA has a low-resistance signal because the brain is a low-resistance vascular bed. The PSV is <125 cm/s, there is a shallow upswing and relatively high EDV.
● The ECA has a high-resistance signal as it supplies a high-resistance vascular bed in the face. There is a sharp systolic upswing and low EDV.
● The CCA signal is a combination of high- and low-resistance signals as flow passes to the two territories.
● Normal vertebral artery signals have PSV $\approx$ 40–60 cm/s with a low-resistance waveform as it supplies the brain.
● Normal subclavian artery signals have PSV $\approx$ 80–150 cm/s with a bi- or triphasic waveform and a prominent reverse component.

Indications for scanning

All patients with cerebrovascular symptoms should have a duplex scan but there is debate as to the value for screening asymptomatic subjects.

Indications include:

● cerebral territory symptoms
● vertebrobasilar insufficiency
● carotid bruit
● a mass in the neck

- pre-operative assessment before aortic aneurysm repair or coronary artery bypass grafting
- surveillance for patients with known stenosis treated conservatively
- surveillance after carotid endarterectomy or stenting.

Lightheadedness, dizziness or non-specific visual disturbances are dubious indications for investigation.

> **Warning!**
>
> Telephone the referring doctor if a symptomatic patient's scan shows 80–99 per cent ICA stenosis.

Criteria for diagnosing disease
Internal carotid artery stenosis

B-mode can accurately determine <50 per cent diameter stenosis but becomes increasingly unreliable for more severe stenosis. Doppler velocities are used to grade >50 per cent diameter stenoses.

We use criteria recommended by the Australasian Society for Ultrasound in Medicine (Table 6.1 and Fig. 6.6). Stenosis is determined by the ratio of internal lumen at the stenosis to lumen in the more distal artery. PSB is present with stenoses >15 per cent.

> **Pitfalls!**
>
> Tortuosity can cause apparent velocity increase even although there is no stenosis. This is due to difficulty in obtaining a correct insonating angle, non-linear or helical flow, or increased velocity on the inside of the curve. Try sampling just beyond the curve.
>
> - There is no agreement as to which of the criteria is most accurate.
> - Ratios are preferred if there are low CCA velocities with reduced cardiac output, or high CCA velocities with high-output cardiac conditions.
> - PSV in the ICA may be increased if there is severe contralateral ICA disease.

Pitfalls!

Trickle flow:

A very tight stenosis causes PSV to fall. If trickle flow is not detected, stenosis may be incorrectly diagnosed as an occlusion. Low-velocity flow can be detected with colour Doppler as a narrow channel in the ICA corresponding to the 'string sign' on arteriography. Power Doppler or contrast imaging help to detect slow flow. Apparent occlusion with ultrasound warrants confirmation by arteriography and the reverse applies for apparent occlusion shown by arteriography.

Table 6.1 Grades of ICA stenosis defined by the Australasian Society for Ultrasound in Medicine

Stenosis	PSV (cm/s)	EDV (cm/s)	Ratio PSV ICA/CCA
16–49%	<125	–	–
50–69%	>125	<110	>2
70–79%	>270	>110	>4
80–99%	>270	>140	>4

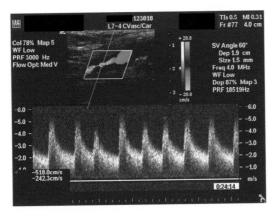

Fig. 6.6

Spectral tracing for 80–99 per cent ICA stenosis.

Stenosis in other carotid arteries

CCA or ECA stenosis is classified as >50 per cent if there is:

- greater than twofold increase in PSV compared with the proximal signal
- delayed systolic upstroke
- post-stenotic turbulence and a dampened distal signal.

Internal carotid artery occlusion

The features are:

- B-mode echoes from occlusive plaque and thrombus throughout the ICA
- no colour or spectral Doppler signal within the ICA
- high-resistance CCA waveform with little, absent or reversed diastolic flow
- low-velocity high-amplitude signal at the ICA origin: 'thump at the stump' (Fig. 6.7)
- meniscus appearance of colour at the ICA origin
- longitudinal pulsations rather than axial expansion of the occluded ICA
- ICA narrowing making it difficult to image if the occlusion is longstanding.

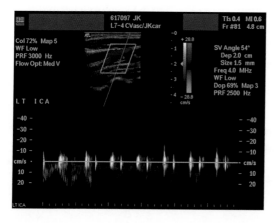

Fig. 6.7

Spectral Doppler showing 'thump at the stump' for ICA occlusion.

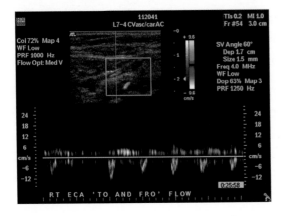

Fig. 6.8

'To-and-fro' flow in the ECA passing to the ICA distal to occlusion of the CCA.

Occlusion in other carotid arteries

A **CCA occlusion** extends from its origin to the bifurcation, may be continuous with an ICA occlusion, and leads to retrograde or 'to-and-fro' flow in the proximal ECA if the ICA is patent (Fig. 6.8).

An **ECA occlusion** is usually segmental over 1–2 cm of the proximal ECA and shows a Doppler signal distal to the occlusion similar to an ICA signal. This can lead to reverse flow or 'to-and-fro' flow in proximal branches feeding the artery beyond the occlusion.

Carotid plaque characteristics

Cerebrovascular events are more often due to emboli from carotid plaque than reduced flow from high-grade stenosis. Plaques are stable or unstable according to their risk of causing embolism (see Chapter 5). Ultrasound assessment of the plaque surface is not very accurate.

Box 6.3: Properties of carotid plaque
Composition and echogenicity
- Homogeneous and hypoechoic
- Heterogeneous and hyperechoic
- Dense calcific with acoustic shadowing

Surface
- Smooth and intact
- Irregular
- Ulcerated

Digital image processing for plaque characterization

Visual assessment of plaque echogenicity and texture is unreliable because it is determined by machine settings and can only be described subjectively. Computer techniques allow quantitative measurement of plaque echogenicity (Fig. 6.9).

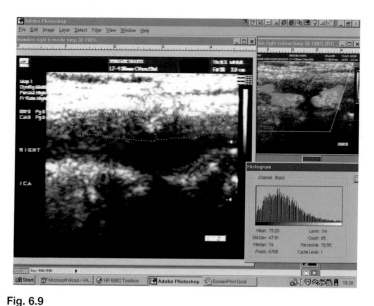

Fig. 6.9

Calculation of carotid plaque echogenicity

- The plaque is defined from the colour Doppler image (above right).
- The plaque outline is drawn with the electronic marker (dashed area of left image).
- Brightness is assessed from low (blood) to high (adventitia) to develop a graph for reference.
- The plaque is digitized for greyscale for all pixels to define a median and standard deviation for echogenicity (lower right inset).

Vertebral artery disease

- There are no established criteria for vertebral artery stenosis.
- A dampened signal suggests proximal vertebral artery disease and a high-resistance signal suggests distal disease.
- Vertebral artery occlusion can only be confirmed if a clear image of the artery is obtained.
- Retrograde flow throughout the cardiac cycle or intermittent forward and reverse ('to-and-fro') flow are indications to examine the subclavian and innominate arteries and to measure systolic pressures in both arms.
- A high-grade ICA stenosis or occlusion can cause increased PSV and diameter in vertebral arteries as they act as collaterals through the circle of Willis.

Subclavian or innominate artery disease

There are no established criteria for grading subclavian artery stenosis but it is reasonable to call a stenosis if the PSV is >200 cm/s with post-stenotic turbulence and a distal dampened signal.

Ultrasound can show characteristic flow direction changes (Table 6.2).

Spectral Doppler shows changes in vertebral arteries (Fig. 6.10).

Table 6.2 Flow directions in extracranial arteries with subclavian or innominate artery stenosis or occlusion

Artery	Disease	R vertebral	L vertebral	R CCA	L CCA
	Normal	↑	↑	N	N
L subclavian	Stenosis	↑	↓ or ↑↓ or ↑	N	N
L subclavian	Occlusion	↑	↓	N	N
R subclavian	Stenosis	↑ or ↑↓ or ↑	↑	N	N
R subclavian	Occlusion	↓	↑	N	N
Innominate	Stenosis	↓ or ↑↓ or ↑	↑	↑	↑↑
Innominate	Occlusion	↓	↑	↑	↑↑

↑: antegrade flow; ↓: retrograde flow; ↑↓: 'to-and-fro' flow; ↑: decreased antegrade flow; N: normal flow; ↑↑: increased flow.

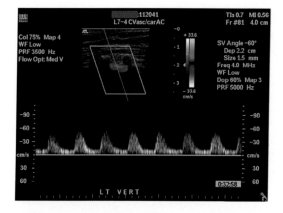

Fig. 6.10

Reverse flow in a vertebral artery due to subclavian artery occlusion.

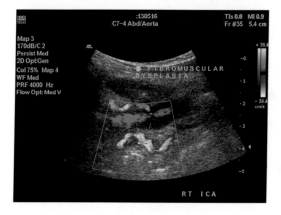

Fig. 6.11

Colour Doppler image of ICA fibromuscular dysplasia

The artery is tortuous with a 'string of beads' appearance due to alternating segments of stenosis and dilatation.

Non-atherosclerotic diseases

Ultrasound may suggest a diagnosis but this almost invariably needs to be confirmed by arteriography and occasionally by arterial biopsy.

- **Fibromuscular dysplasia** shows tortuosity and dilatations in the mid to distal extracranial ICA just as for the renal arteries (Fig. 6.11).
- **Carotid artery dissection** shows a long, narrow residual lumen through the length of the ICA (Fig. 6.12) or ICA occlusion.
- **Carotid aneurysms** show distal CCA and proximal ICA dilatation associated with mural thrombus.

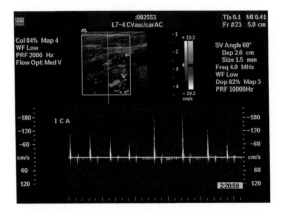

Fig. 6.12

Spectral Doppler tracing of an ICA dissection

There is a limited sharp pulse due to relative obstruction. If the artery is still patent, there may be multiple sites of entry and exit of flow.

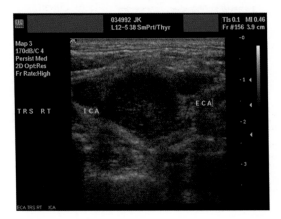

Fig. 6.13

B-mode of carotid body tumour in transverse showing splaying of the ICA and ECA by the tumour mass.

- **Carotid body tumour** shows a mass on B-mode that splays the carotid bifurcation to cause a 'saddle appearance' (Fig. 6.13), and colour Doppler shows it to be highly vascular, fed by branches from the ECA.
- **Takayasu's disease** shows highly specific homogeneous circumferential intima–media thickening of the CCA on B-mode.
- **Temporal arteritis** frequently shows a characteristic 'halo' appearance on B-mode or colour Doppler due to peri-adventitial oedema, and this typically disappears after treatment with steroids.

● **Moya-Moya syndrome** is associated with extensive arterial occlusions or high-grade stenoses of extracranial carotid and vertebral arteries with a rich collateral circulation.

PROTOCOLS FOR SCANNING

Follow scanning techniques discussed on page 38 in Chapter 2. Always scan both sides.

Prepare the patient

Read the referral and question the patient. Think about symptoms and predict the site of disease. It can be difficult to communicate with a patient with stroke causing deficits that affect speech, movement, memory, or even consciousness.

Note!

ICA disease can cause contralateral motor or sensory symptoms or ipsilateral amaurosis fugax.

Select the best transducer

● Use the linear array transducer to image extracranial arteries.
● Use the curved array transducer to scan a patient with a bull neck or to image the distal ICA.
● Use the phased array transducer with its small footprint to study arch branches, angling from above the clavicle medially and inferiorly, and to study the distal ICA through the submandibular window just below the angle of the jaw.

Carotid arteries

Position the patient and select a window

● Lie the patient supine if possible. Position yourself sitting either behind the head (Fig. 6.14) or facing the patient.

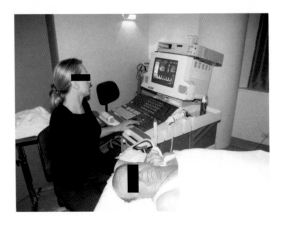

Fig. 6.14

Our preferred position for scanning carotid arteries.

- Turn the head 45° away from the side being examined with the chin tilted upwards. Use one flat pillow or no pillow to extend the neck.
- Vary the angle of approach or patient head position as required.
- Move the transducer to where arteries are most superficial.
- Image through the sternomastoid muscle or internal jugular vein rather than fat.
- Use a posteromedial window for the distal ICA to avoid interference by the mandible.
- Examine the carotid bifurcation from medial, anterior and posteromedial windows to find one that may counteract back-shadowing by calcified plaque.
- Use the submandibular window to show the more distal retromandibular and extradural ICA. This is useful to detect ICA dissections or fibromuscular dysplasia.

Tips!

- Begin each scan on the same side, usually the right.
- Avoid excess pressure on the carotid bifurcation that may stimulate the carotid sinus to cause bradycardia, syncope or even ventricular asystole.
- Avoid excess pressure that can compress arteries to cause spurious high velocities.

Scanning techniques for carotid arteries

Box 6.4: It is vital to distinguish the ICA from the ECA

Image the arteries by B-mode to observe the:

- ICA has a larger diameter than the ECA near the bifurcation
- ECA is anteromedial to the ICA at the bifurcation
- ICA usually then runs posterior to the ECA (but not always).

Use colour Doppler to show the:

- artery with branches is the ECA.

Use spectral Doppler to show:

- the ICA has a low-resistance waveform (high EDV) and the ECA a high-resistance waveform (low EDV)
- lightly tapping the superficial temporal artery in front of the ear produces a saw-tooth pattern in the ECA waveform: the tap test requires practice and the image should be interpreted with caution in inexperienced hands.

- In B-mode, image carotid arteries in transverse from the clavicle to mandible with special attention to the carotid bifurcation, noting the relation of the ICA to the ECA. Note the position, extent and type of plaque and measure diameters of the ICA, ECA and distal CCA.
- Use colour Doppler to image the CCA, ICA and proximal ECA in longitudinal, noting areas of aliasing and lumen narrowing.
- Obtain spectral Doppler signals in the CCA, ICA and proximal ECA and any areas of suspected stenosis, noting the PSV, EDV and presence or absence of spectral broadening.
- Note if there is tortuosity, as this is a differential diagnosis as a cause for bruit and is also important to record prior to carotid endarterectomy.

> ## Tips!
>
> ● Disease is most common in the carotid bulb so 'walk' a Doppler sample volume from the distal CCA through the proximal ICA to be sure to detect stenoses.
> ● Normal boundary layer separation within the carotid bulb is a reassuring sign that there is no stenosis.

How to distinguish severe stenosis from occlusion

To detect trickle flow:

● reduce the colour velocity range to a minimum
● steer the colour box straight
● use the venous scanning setup for low flow: low PRF and low wall filter
● increase colour persistence
● reduce the angle of insonation
● use spectral Doppler as it is more sensitive than colour Doppler. All occlusions must be confirmed by spectral Doppler
● increase the Doppler sample volume to cover the entire lumen
● change to a higher frequency transducer
● consider power Doppler which is very sensitive to low flow.

Vertebral arteries

Position the patient and select a window

Vertebral arteries can be imaged from their origins to mid-cervical region. Straighten the patient's head and use an anterior or lateral approach. It can be difficult to see flow in vertebral arteries; if so, then decrease the colour scale, try different windows and turn the head to the side.

Scanning techniques for vertebral arteries

● Show the CCA and then find the vertebral artery just lateral and posterior identified by its path through dark 'shadowed' areas of the spinous processes.

● Use colour Doppler to identify the vertebral artery
● Assess with spectral Doppler to look for flow direction, PSV and type of resistance. What appears to be reverse flow may be due to tortuosity or flow in the adjacent vertebral vein.

Arch branches

Position the patient and select a window

Turn the patient's head away from the side you are scanning. Use the small-footprint phased array transducer to angle over the clavicle if necessary.

Scanning techniques for arch branches

● Examine each subclavian artery from its origin and obtain a spectral trace and PSV in a suspected stenosis.
● Plaque can often be seen using B-mode or a filling defect with colour Doppler.
● Record brachial systolic pressures in both arms if subclavian or innominate artery disease is suspected. A difference >20 mmHg shows that there is significant disease.

Box 6.5: Ultrasound images to record

● B-mode in longitudinal of the proximal CCA, carotid bifurcation and ICA.
● B-mode of significant plaque in transverse and longitudinal (colour Doppler if plaque is echolucent).
● Sample spectral traces of the proximal and distal CCA, proximal and distal ICA, proximal ECA, vertebral and subclavian arteries.
● Spectral trace in any area of stenosis or occlusion.
● Other lesions or non-atherosclerotic pathology.

7

TRANSCRANIAL DOPPLER AND DUPLEX ULTRASOUND SCANNING

Ultrasound can be used to study intracranial arteries through 'windows' where bone is thin or absent. The original technique of transcranial Doppler (TCD) uses dedicated pulsed-Doppler to show spectral analysis alone. A duplex scanner can be used for transcranial colour Doppler (TCCD). TCCD can visualize arteries for correct identification but does not insonate vessels as well as TCD. Either can detect pathological variations, flow abnormalities or embolic signals in patients with vasospasm from subarachnoid haemorrhage, extracranial or intracranial arterial disease, stroke or head injury. Both are simple, non-invasive and inexpensive but angiography is required for more comprehensive anatomical detail.

ANATOMY

Box 7.1: Arteries scanned for reporting
- Internal carotid artery: ICA
- Vertebral artery
- Basilar artery
- Anterior cerebral artery: ACA

- Middle cerebral artery: MCA
- Posterior cerebral artery: PCA
- Anterior communicating artery: ACoA
- Posterior communicating artery: PCoA

Other arteries discussed

- External carotid artery: ECA
- Anterior and posterior inferior cerebellar arteries: AICA and PICA

Arteries of the cerebral circulation join at the base of brain as the circle of Willis (Fig. 7.1). Circulation to the anterior brain is from the ICA, and its intracranial portion commences in the carotid canal at the base of skull (Fig. 7.2). There are connections between branches of the ICA and ECA (Fig. 7.3). Circulation to the posterior brain is from the vertebral arteries and basilar artery (Fig. 7.4).

Clinical aspects

Regional pathology and clinical presentations

Vasospasm from subarachnoid haemorrhage

This is usually due to bleeding from an intracranial aneurysm and is the most frequent indication for TCD or TCCD in many services. Vasospasm can lead to secondary cerebral ischaemia and tends to develop at about three days after haemorrhage, peaks at one week, and disappears within two weeks. Serial TCD or TCCD help to determine whether medical treatment is required for vasospasm and when it is safe to stop treatment.

Intracranial arterial disease

TCD or TCCD shows that intracranial cerebral arterial stenosis due to atherosclerosis can reduce perfusion and disturb cerebral autoregulation and vasomotor reactivity. Small vessel damage can result from hypertension, diabetes or arteritis causing increased peripheral resistance.

Extracranial arterial disease

Extracranial ICA stenosis or occlusion can reduce blood flow in intracranial arteries leading to collateral circulation through the circle

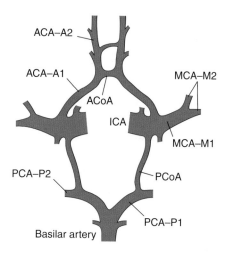

Fig. 7.1

Circle of Willis

- Carotid and vertebrobasilar systems communicate from side to side and front to back.
- The ACoA connects the ACAs.
- Each PCoA connects the PCA and MCA on that side.
- Each ACA passes medially then superiorly between the frontal lobes:
  - A1: segment before the ACoA
  - A2: segment after the ACoA.
- Each MCA passes horizontally and laterally and then bifurcates or trifurcates into branches:
  - M1: segment before branching
  - M2: segment after branching.
- Each PCA passes forwards and laterally, then laterally and posteriorly:
  - P1: segment before the PCoA
  - P2: segment after the PCoA.
- One or more segments of the circle are absent in 50 per cent, most often with hypoplasia of the PCoA, so that potential collateral circulation can be deficient.
- The PCA arises directly from the ICA, replacing the PCoA in 15 per cent.

Redrawn from Lord, RSA. 1986: *Surgery of Occlusive Cerebrovascular Disease*. St Louis: CV Mosby. By kind permission of the author.

of Willis. Autoregulation reduces peripheral resistance to compensate for decreased perfusion to a critical point before ischaemia develops. It is usual to treat high-grade extracranial ICA stenosis by carotid endarterectomy (see page 103 in Chapter 6).

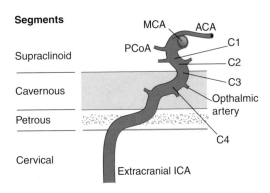

Fig. 7.2

Intracranial ICA

- Passes through the foramen lacerum in the temporal bone.
- Carotid siphon forms an S-shape curving forwards then backwards.
- ICA forms four segments.
- Gives branches including the ophthalmic artery and PCoA.
- Bifurcates into the smaller ACA and larger MCA.

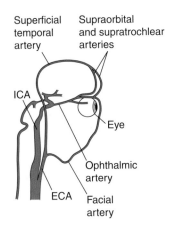

Fig. 7.3

Periorbital circulation with connections between the ICA and ECA through the orbit

- The ophthalmic artery passes forward through the optic canal to supply the eye.
- It gives supraorbital and supratrochlear branches that anastomose with facial and superficial temporal branches of the ECA.

Fig. 83 from Rumwell C and McPharlin M 1996: *Vascular Technology*. Pasadena: Davies Publishers. Reproduced with permission.

Stroke from cerebral infarction

Stroke is due to extracranial disease causing embolism or secondary thrombosis in intracranial arteries in more than two-thirds of patients. Stroke results from intracranial occlusive disease alone in approximately 20 per cent or from intracranial haemorrhage in the

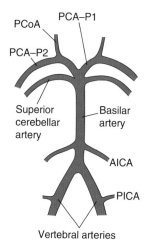

Fig. 7.4

Vertebrobasilar arteries

- Vertebral arteries pass anteriorly and medially to enter the cranium through the foramen magnum.
- They join to form the basilar artery which passes anteriorly and superiorly to its bifurcation into the PCAs.
- Branches include the cerebellar arteries.
- The pathway of the vertebral arteries is variable.

remainder. An acute stroke can lead to loss of autoregulation in adjacent brain tissue that can take two weeks to recover.

Head injury

Further damage after brain trauma results from cerebral ischaemia due to intracranial hypertension causing disturbed autoregulation and decreased blood flow. Serial TCD or TCCD can detect reduced perfusion and monitor the effect of medical treatment.

Cerebral microemboli

Fibrin and platelet aggregates produce characteristic random high-intensity transient signals (HITS) on TCD or TCCD as they pass through intracranial arteries. Many hours of monitoring may be required to detect HITS, although automated systems are now available to store results.

Conditions associated with HITS include:

- extracranial arterial disease
- atrial fibrillation
- prosthetic cardiac valves
- cerebral angiography
- left ventricular catheterization
- decompression illness

- fat embolism
- cardiopulmonary bypass
- carotid endarterectomy.

They are more common and numerous in patients with symptomatic ICA disease. They can cause silent strokes that lead to cognitive impairment after coronary artery bypass surgery. More than 50 HITS per hour detected during and after carotid endarterectomy strongly predict peri-operative neurological deficits.

What the doctors need to know

There is still debate about the relevance of information obtained.

- **Carotid endarterectomy.** TCD or TCCD can show changes before, during and after operation that might influence technique and follow-up care.
- **Diagnosis and monitoring in the intensive care unit.** A single study is frequently requested to assess the effects of stroke or head injury. Serial studies can monitor cerebral perfusion and guide treatment after subarachnoid haemorrhage.
- **Treatment after stroke.** TCD or TCCD can show intracranial stenosis, occlusion or acute thrombosis, and this might influence whether to give antiplatelet, anticoagulation or thrombolytic therapy.

TRANSCRANIAL DOPPLER AND DUPLEX SCANNING

TCD provides no anatomical detail but usually gives spectral tracings for most arteries studied. TCCD gives more information but it is unusual to see all arteries. In practice, it is reasonable to start with TCCD then move on to TCD if it is available. It is not possible to image through bone in approximately 10 per cent of patients. Ultrasound contrast agents or power Doppler improve sensitivity.

Box 7.2: Abbreviations
- PSV: peak systolic velocity
- EDV: end diastolic volume
- PI: pulsatility index

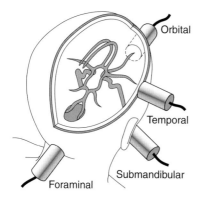

Fig. 7.5

Windows for TCD or TCCD

Redrawn from Fig. 36.1 Bernstein EF. 1993: *Vascular Diagnosis*. St Louis: CV Mosby. With permission of the publisher.

Windows for TCD and TCCD

TCD and TCCD require 'windows' where bone is thin or absent (Fig. 7.5).

Normal findings

Box 7.3: Calculations

Mean velocity = (PSV − EDV)/3 + EDV

PI = (PSV − EDV)/mean velocity

Haemodynamic index = mean velocity MCA/mean velocity ICA (if studying vasospasm)

Mean velocities are preferred to PSV or EDV since they are less affected by systemic haemodynamic factors such as heart rate and contractility or peripheral resistance. There is a broad range of mean velocities for various arteries (Table 7.1) and velocities decrease with advancing age. PI is variable.

● Velocities can vary appreciably so that abnormal flow may be detected more accurately if there is a difference in mean velocity between each side.
● Many arteries show flow almost directly towards or away from the transducer and this gives maximum Doppler shifts with a small error even for 15–20° variations in insonation angles. TCCD allows for angle correction.

Table 7.1 Normal mean velocities, artery depth form transducer, flow direction and window from ATL (Advanced Technology Ltd) criteria.

Artery	Mean velocity (cm/s)	Depth from transducer (mm)	Flow direction to transducer	Window
MCA (M1)	62 ± 12	40–60	Towards	Temporal
ACA (A1)	50 ± 12	65–75	Away	Temporal
ICA	Varies	65	Towards	Temporal
Ophthalmic	20 ± 10	45–65	Towards	Orbital
PCA (P1)	42 ± 10	65–75	Towards	Temporal
PCA (P2)	40 ± 10	60–70	Away	Temporal
Vertebral	36 ± 10	60–85	Away	Foraminal
Basilar	39 ± 10	>85	Away	Foraminal

- Turbulence is not normally observed. Doppler shifts from the ICA are considerably lower than those in the ACA and MCA owing to more oblique insonation. Flow is not detected if there is congenital or acquired absence of a segment in the circle of Willis.
- There can be appreciable flow variations depending on mental or physical activity.

Indications for TCD or TCCD

- Tight stenosis or occlusion of the ICA or CCA.
- Concern as to the presence of intracranial arterial disease.
- Transient ischaemic attacks with no other source of embolism.
- Vertebral artery disease.
- Arterial noises in the ear.
- Syncope or dizziness with head rotation.
- Monitoring cerebral perfusion in the intensive care unit after stroke, subarachnoid haemorrhage or head injury.
- Studying changes in intracranial haemodynamics and emboli during carotid endarterectomy or coronary artery bypass grafting.

Criteria for diagnosing disease

Vasospasm or intracranial stenosis

TCD and TCCD show characteristic findings provided that systemic haemodynamic parameters are kept constant:

- absolute increase in mean velocity in the MCA:
  - minor: 120–150cm/s

- moderate: 150–200 cm/s
- severe: >200 cm/s
- a ≥50 per cent velocity increase above preliminary baseline values, or side-to-side mean velocity difference ≥35 per cent for the MCA
- increased haemodynamic index due to impaired autoregulation. Calculation of the index requires measurement of velocities in the ICA from the cervical view or submandibular window:
  - minor: 3–5
  - moderate: 5–7
  - severe: >7.

Occlusive arterial disease

This may cause decreased mean velocity, reduced PI, and reduced cerebrovascular reactivity. HITS are more likely to be demonstrated.

Carotid artery and vertebrobasilar disease

TCD and TCCD show characteristic changes for flow-reducing ICA stenosis or occlusion (Fig. 7.6) and basilar artery occlusion (Fig. 7.7).

Subclavian steal syndrome

TCD and TCCD may demonstrate flow changes in the ipsilateral vertebral artery and intracranial arteries in patients with subclavian steal (Fig. 7.8). Lesser degrees of disease cause spectral deceleration, and more severe disease causes alternating or 'to-and-fro' flow (see page 109 in Chapter 6). In borderline cases, stress testing by arm exercise may induce flow changes.

Stroke

TCD or TCCD help differentiate reasons for stroke:

- lack of collateral pathways, low MCA velocity, reduced MCA PI and reduced vasomotor reactivity favour haemodynamic insufficiency
- apparent major branch occlusion suggests artery-to-artery embolism if extracranial disease has been demonstrated

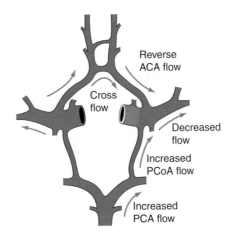

Fig. 7.6

TCD and TCCD changes with a right ICA occlusion or tight stenosis

- Reduced mean velocity in the ipsilateral MCA, absolute or relative to the other side.
- Low PI in the ipsilateral MCA from increased diastolic velocity due to distal vasodilatation.
- Decreased or reversed ipsilateral ACA flow and increased contralateral ACA flow causing side-to-side difference of mean velocities ⩾30 per cent.
- Collateral flow across the ACoA.
- Increased collateral flow in the ipsilateral PCoA.
- Increased velocity in the ipsilateral PCA causing side-to-side difference of mean velocities ⩾20 per cent.
- Retrograde flow in the ipsilateral ophthalmic artery.

- normal TCD or TCCD studies in a patient with likely embolic stroke suggest the heart as a possible source.

Head injury

A mean velocity ⩽35 cm/s in one or both MCAs with a high ipsilateral PI is associated with a poor prognosis.

Brain death

Increasing brain damage in the process of dying results in a greatly increased PI with loss of forward flow and then reverse flow in diastole.

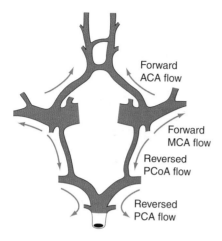

Fig. 7.7

TCD and TCCD changes with basilar artery occlusion or tight stenosis

Reverse flow in PCoA and PCA.

Forward ACA flow

Forward MCA flow

Reversed PCoA flow

Reversed PCA flow

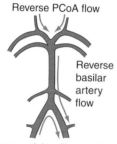

Reverse PCoA flow

Reverse basilar artery flow

Increase right vertebral artery flow

Reverse left vertebral artery flow

Fig. 7.8

Possible TCD or TCCD changes for subclavian steal

Left subclavian artery occlusion may cause:

- reverse flow in the left vertebral artery
- increased antegrade flow in the right vertebral artery
- reverse flow in the basilar artery and PCoAs.

Carotid endarterectomy

While deciding whether to advise surgery, TCD or TCCD can show whether there is:

- normal or reduced ipsilateral perfusion
- tandem intracranial disease
- normal or reduced cross-flow through the circle of Willis.

During and after carotid endarterectomy, TCD or TCCD can show:

- cerebral perfusion during occlusion from carotid clamping to select patients requiring shunting
- HITS.

Cerebral microembolism

Features that distinguish HITS from artefacts are signals that are:

- 4 dB above the background erythrocyte spectrum
- unidirectional and not crossing the baseline
- of short duration <20 ms
- a random occurrence.

PROTOCOLS FOR TCD AND TCCD

Prepare the patient

It may be difficult for a patient to understand the subtle reasons for the investigation. Explain the procedure and address safety concerns. Studies can be difficult in an unconscious patient. Provocative tests that can be used to increase flow and test vasomotor reactivity include hyperventilation or breathing 6 per cent CO_2. Head rotation can be used to kink vertebral arteries.

Select the best transducer

The dedicated pulsed-Doppler system for TCD has a frequency of 2–3 MHz. A small-footprint 2 MHz phased array transducer is required for TCCD.

Obtain the optimal image

If no flow is detected by TCD or TCCD, the reasons could be:

- poor study for TCCD
- poor window or the bone too thick
- arterial calcification or occlusion
- unfavourable insonation angle
- anatomical variations or vessel tortuosity
- velocity range too high
- low flow velocity or volume
- wall filter set too high
- gain or power set too low.

Optimize B-mode

- **Frame rate:** increase to improve temporal resolution.
- **Dynamic range:** adjust to provide more contrast (low dynamic range) and easier vessel identification.

Optimize colour Doppler

Colour helps to place the sample volume, detect increased flow by aliasing and turbulence.

- **Colour gain:** set high to show low flow.
- **Wall filter:** set high to eliminate wall motion artefact.
- **Colour velocity range:** adjust for low velocities.
- **Frame rate:** keep as high as possible.

Optimize spectral Doppler

- **Spectral direction:** show flow towards the transducer above the baseline.
- **Baseline:** centre to demonstrate bidirectional flow then lower if there are high velocities.
- **Sample volume size:** increase size if it is difficult to record a signal.
- **Wall filter:** set moderately high to eliminate wall motion noise.
- **Doppler gain:** adjust to fill the spectral waveform without causing artefactual mirroring.

Pitfalls!

- There may be a poor acoustic window.
- There is a relatively narrow field of view.
- Only a short segment of each artery is seen.
- It requires a clear signal to measure mean velocities.
- TCD measurements assume a zero angle and this is rarely correct.
- It is necessary to determine which vessel is being studied from its depth.
- Anatomy is highly variable.
- Branches can be confusing.
- It is frequently not possible to distinguish tight stenosis from occlusion.

Temporal window

The temporal bone is thin in young patients but becomes thicker with increasing age, especially in females.

Position the patient and select the window

The patient lies supine with the head upright to allow scanning from the side. Scan both right and left sides. Place the transducer above the zygomatic arch in front of the ear. Several positions are available (Fig. 7.9) but usually only one gives a clear image.

Scanning techniques for temporal window

This shows arterial branches of the ICA circulation as well as the PCA (Fig. 7.10).

The arteries are insonated with the transducer held in transverse and the image orientation marker anteriorly.

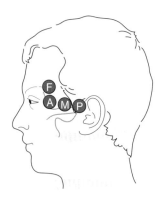

Fig. 7.9

Temporal views

- F: Frontal window over the thin frontal bone.
- A: Anterior temporal window behind the frontal process of the zygoma.
- M: Middle temporal window.
- P: Posterior temporal pre-auricular window.

Redrawn from Fig. 36.3 Bernstein EF. 1993: *Vascular Diagnosis*. St Louis: CV Mosby. By kind permission from CV Mosby.

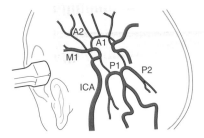

Fig. 7.10

Temporal window

Redrawn from Blackburn D and Jones A. 1994: *ATL Vascular Duplex Protocol Guides*. Washington: Site Bothell. Reproduced with permission from the authors.

- The ICA can be insonated from the cavernous sinus to its bifurcation.
- There is bidirectional flow at the bifurcation into MCA and ACA (Fig. 7.11).
- The M1 segment to the MCA bifurcation is pointed directly at the transducer.
- The M2 segment can usually be insonated.
- The P1 segment is best seen close to the midline between the basilar artery bifurcation and PCoA.
- The PCoA is only seen if it is a major collateral with severe ICA disease.

Techniques are similar for TCD and TCCD:

- use ample gel. Move the transducer slowly in small steps taking care to maintain good contact. Use only moderate pressure to avoid discomfort
- identify bony landmarks with B-mode. Angle the transducer inferiorly to identify the sphenoid and petrous ridges (Fig. 7.12)

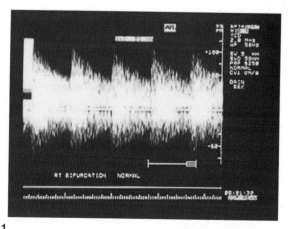

Fig. 7.11

TCD at the ICA bifurcation showing bidirectional flow into the ACA and MCA

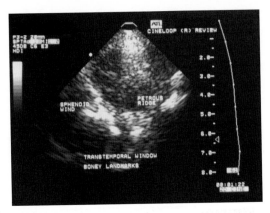

Fig. 7.12

Temporal view for TCCD

Angle the transducer inferiorly to show the sphenoid and petrous temporal ridges.

- show the arteries with colour and spectral Doppler for TCCD (Fig. 7.13). Spectral analysis provides the most useful information:
  - the ACoA and PCoA are usually not seen unless acting as collaterals
  - anterior circulation arteries are to the left and posterior circulation arteries to the right of the screen
  - the ipsilateral MCA is closest to the transducer, the ipsilateral ACA and PCA are in the mid-field and the corresponding contralateral arteries are furthest away
- focus to the appropriate depth to find each artery
- tilt the transducer horizontally and vertically to search for the arteries. Use fine adjustments to obtain the best images
- identify each artery by showing its relative position and flow direction to the transducer. The main landmark is where the ICA branches into the ACA and MCA.

Foraminal window

Position the patient and select the window

Flex the head with the chin down to the chest to open the gap between the cranium and atlas.

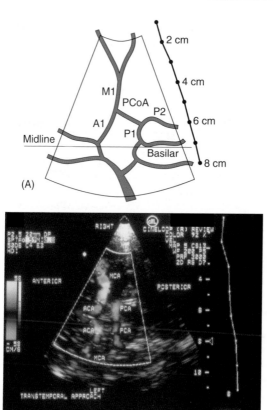

Fig. 7.13

Temporal view for TCCD

Angle the transducer superiorly to insonate the arteries.
A: Diagram of the anatomy.
B: Colour Doppler image.

Scanning techniques for foraminal window

This shows the vertebral arteries, and proximal and middle segments of the basilar artery (Fig. 7.14).

Hold the transducer in transverse with the orientation marker to the left.

● The vertebral arteries are seen just lateral to the midline. They run a variable course.

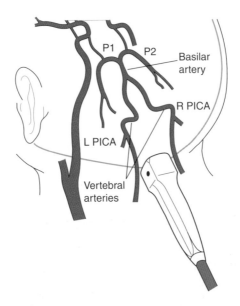

Fig. 7.14

Foraminal window

Redrawn from Blackburn D and Jones A. 1994: *ATL Vascular Duplex Protocol Guides.* Washington: Site Bothell. Reproduced with permission from the authors.

- The basilar artery produces a signal in the midline at a deeper level.
- There is a change in Doppler shift at the vertebrobasilar junction with TCD.
- Signals from the PICA can be seen with flow towards the transducer.

Place the transducer in the midline and direct the beam forwards and then slightly to each side (Fig. 7.15).

Orbital window

Position the patient and select the window

The patient lies supine. Lower the power to 10 per cent to insonate through the orbital window thereby reducing ultrasonic exposure to the eye.

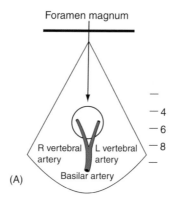

(A)

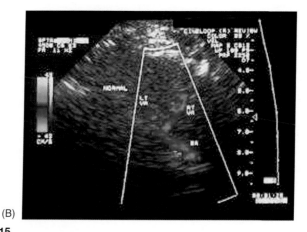

(B)

Fig. 7.15

Foraminal view for TCCD

A: Diagram of the anatomy.
B: Colour Doppler image.

Scanning techniques for orbital window

This shows the carotid siphon and ophthalmic artery (Fig. 7.16). C2 flow is away from and C4 flow is towards the transducer.

Scan with the transducer held in transverse and orientation marker to the left.

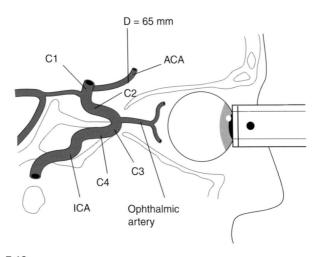

Fig. 7.16

Orbital window

Fig. 7 from Aaslid R. 1986: *Transcranial Doppler Sonography*. Vienna: Springer-Verlag. Reproduced by kind permission of Springer-Verlag.

● Remove contact lenses prior to the examination.
● Angle slightly off centre to avoid insonating through the lens to the retina.
● Place the transducer over the closed eyelid with ample gel applied. It is not necessary to put pressure on the transducer to maintain good contact.
● Explore different positions to obtain the best image.
● The ophthalmic artery points towards the transducer.
● Progressively increasing the depth brings the carotid siphon into view.
● In some cases, the ACA can be insonated through the thin orbital roof.

Submandibular window

Insonating upwards from below the mandible shows the distal ICA as it approaches the carotid canal. It complements extracranial studies. It is particularly useful to show ICA dissection and chronic occlusion with restoration of flow through ECA collaterals.

Box 7.4: Ultrasound images to record

For each window:

- colour Doppler of arteries
- spectral trace for each artery listed in Box 7.1 for PSV, EDV and flow direction relative to the transducer
- calculate PI and mean velocity from PSV and EDV for each artery
- if studying for vasospasm, calculate haemodynamic index from PSV and EDV in ICA and MCA.

8

DISEASES OF ARTERIES TO THE LOWER LIMBS

Duplex scanning can determine the location, extent and type of occlusive or aneurysmal disease. For occlusive disease, ankle to brachial arterial pressure indices can screen for disease, and ultrasound is then commonly used to plan clinical treatment. With aneurysms, ultrasound is used for screening and surveillance, but computed tomography more accurately measures size while arteriography is required in selected patients.

ANATOMY

Box 8.1: Arteries scanned for reporting

- Abdominal aorta
- Common iliac artery: CIA
- Internal iliac artery: IIA
- External iliac artery: EIA
- Common femoral artery: CFA
- Profunda femoris artery: PFA
- Superficial femoral artery: SFA
- Popliteal artery
- Tibioperoneal trunk
- Posterior tibial artery: PTA
- Anterior tibial artery: ATA
- Peroneal artery

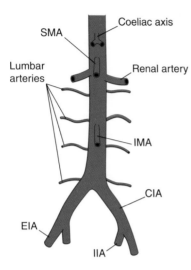

Fig. 8.1

Abdominal aorta

- Lies to the left of midline with the inferior vena cava to its right.
- Extends from L1 to L4 vertebrae.
- Gives visceral branches.
- Also gives phrenic and lumbar parietal branches.

Ultrasound can study arteries from the diaphragm to the feet (Figs 8.1–8.4).

CLINICAL ASPECTS: OCCLUSIVE DISEASE

Regional pathology

Occlusive disease is usually caused by atherosclerosis and is usually segmental rather than diffuse. Stenosis results from atheromatous plaques (Fig. 8.5, page 146). Occlusion is caused by plaques and secondary thrombosis between branches that supply collaterals. Common sites are the full length of the infrarenal

---

Box 8.2: Sites for disease

The approximate frequency for predominant disease at each level is:

- aortoiliac ≈25 per cent
- femoropopliteal ≈65 per cent
- infrapopliteal ≈10 per cent, more frequent in diabetics.

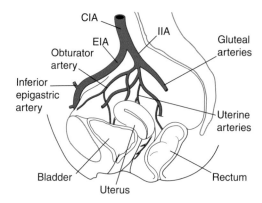

Fig. 8.2

Iliac arteries (female)

Each CIA:

- extends from L4 to the sacroiliac joint
- is 4–5 cm long
- divides into the IIA and EIA
- lies to the left of the corresponding common iliac vein.

Each EIA:

- is approximately twice the length of the CIA
- lies superficial to the corresponding vein
- gives the inferior epigastric artery passing upwards and anterior just above the inguinal ligament
- becomes the CFA at the inguinal ligament.

aorta, CIA or EIA since each usually has small or no branches (Fig. 8.6, page 147). Infrainguinal occlusions can affect the SFA between two large muscular branches, or the popliteal artery and crural arteries (Fig. 8.7, page 148). There may be multiple occlusions with isolated patent segments in between (Fig. 8.8, page 149).

Clinical presentations

The severity of symptoms (Fig. 8.9, page 149) depends on:

- which arteries are involved
- the extent and number of lesions
- whether there is stenosis or occlusion
- the extent of collaterals.

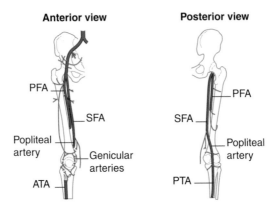

Anterior view   **Posterior view**

Fig. 8.3

Femoral and popliteal arteries

Each CFA:

- lies superficially in the groin
- is 4–6 cm long
- divides to form the SFA and PFA.

Each SFA:

- extends down the medial thigh
- passes deep through the hiatus of the adductor magnus muscle.

Each popliteal artery:

- commences below the adductor hiatus
- passes vertically through the popliteal fossa
- divides to form the tibioperoneal trunk and ATA.

The patient is examined for the appearance of the legs and feet. The femoral, popliteal, posterior tibial and dorsalis pedis pulses are palpated to determine if they are normal, reduced or absent.
A stethoscope detects bruits over the upper and mid abdomen, inguinal region, adductor hiatus, and popliteal fossa.

Intermittent claudication

Characteristic features are:

- reproducible muscle pain with exercise
- alternatively, fatigue, heaviness or tightness with exercise

Anterior view   **Posterior view**

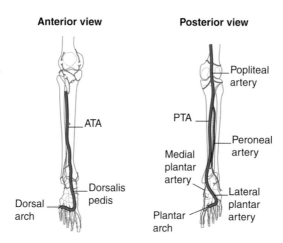

Fig. 8.4

Crural arteries

- The tibioperoneal trunk divides to form the PTA and peroneal artery.
- The ATA passes anterior to the tibia to supply the anterior compartment and continues as the dorsalis pedis artery in the foot.
- The PTA runs posterior to the tibia to supply the back of calf and continues as the plantar arteries in the foot.
- The peroneal artery runs medial to the fibula to supply the deep compartment.
- There are several interconnections so that each can supply all regions.

- walking distance reduced on an incline
- distance to claudication constant
- relief by rest for 3–5 min.

Claudication may be limited to the calf with disease at any level. Pain in the calf and thigh always indicates disease proximal to the SFA, and buttock claudication indicates disease in the aorta, CIAs or IIAs. Occasionally, claudication is isolated to the buttock with IIA disease, the thigh with PFA disease, or the foot with crural artery disease.

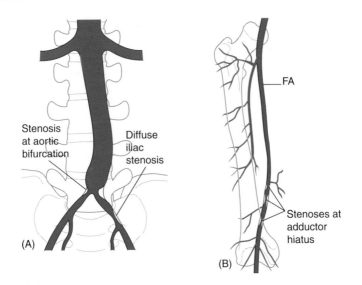

Fig. 8.5

Lower limb arterial stenoses

Common sites are:

A: at the aortic bifurcation extending through the iliac arteries

B: in the SFA at the adductor hiatus.

Fig. 12.1e and f from Myers KA, Marshall RD and Freidin J. 1980: *Principles of Pathology*. Oxford: Blackwell. Reproduced with permission from Blackwell.

The Leriche syndrome

Occlusion of the abdominal aorta can cause (Rene Leriche, (1879–1955), a French surgeon):

- buttock, thigh and calf claudication
- impotence
- diminished or absent femoral pulses.

Critical ischaemia

More severe ischaemia is commonly caused by disease at multiple levels.

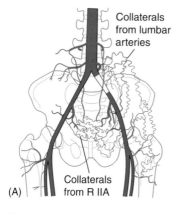
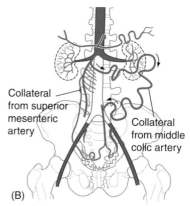

Fig. 8.6

Aortic and iliac artery occlusions

A: CIA occlusion: collaterals

- arise from parietal arteries and
- pass to IIA and PFA branches.

B: Aortic occlusion: collaterals

- arise from visceral arteries and
- pass to IIA branches.

Fig. 12.16a and b from Myers KA, Marshall RD and Freidin J. 1980: *Principles of Pathology*. Oxford: Blackwell. Reproduced with permission from Blackwell.

- Rest pain particularly occurs at night.
- Ischaemic ulceration can develop over pressure points or sites of trauma.
- Gangrene (infarction with secondary putrefaction) usually affects the toes but can occur on the heel or anterior tibial compartment.
- Multiple small emboli can cause the 'blue toe syndrome'.

Differential diagnosis

If leg pain is not clearly associated with exercise but occurs with standing, sitting or lying down then consider:

- sciatica or other neurogenic causes
- spinal canal stenosis
- arthritis

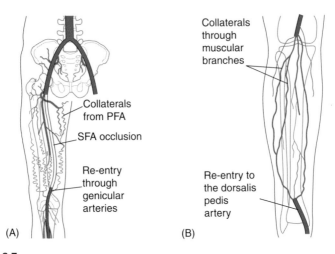

Fig. 8.7

Infrainguinal arterial occlusions

A: SFA occlusion: collaterals

- arise from PFA and SFA branches and
- pass to genicular arteries at the knee.

B: Popliteal and crural artery occlusion: collaterals

- arise from genicular arteries and
- pass through muscular branches to reform distal crural arteries.

Figs 12.16d and 12.17b from Myers KA, Marshall RD and Freidin J. 1980: *Principles of Pathology*. Oxford: Blackwell. Reproduced with permission from Blackwell.

- musculoskeletal causes
- venous claudication.

Treatment

There are various options according to the severity of disease (Fig. 8.10).

Disease commonly involves more than one arterial segment and it can be difficult to assess the relative contribution from each. Symptoms are not relieved if the wrong segment is treated.

Conservative management

Most patients with intermittent claudication are advised to continue walking despite pain and modify risk factors for atherosclerosis,

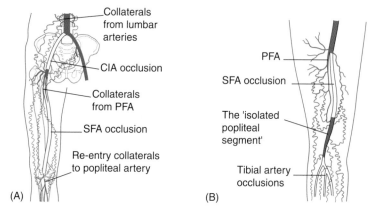

(A) (B)

Fig. 8.8

Multiple arterial occlusions

A: CIA and SFA occlusions: collaterals

- arise from parietal and visceral arteries and IIA branches
- re-enter the isolated CFA segment
- pass from PFA branches through the genicular arteries to the popliteal artery.

B: SFA and crural artery occlusions: collaterals

- arise from branches of the PFA
- re-enter the isolated popliteal segment
- pass from the genicular arteries to muscular branches to the leg.

Figs 12.16i and 12.17a from Myers KA, Marshall RD and Freidin J. 1980: *Principles of Pathology*. Oxford: Blackwell. Reproduced with permission from Blackwell.

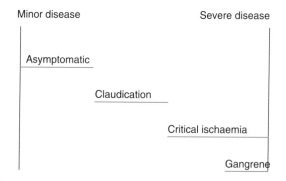

Fig. 8.9

The range of clinical presentations

Fig. 8.3 from Myers KA, Sumner DS and Nicolaides AN. 1997: *Lower Limb Ischaemia*. London: Medorion.

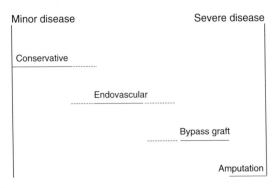

Fig. 8.10

Different doctors have varying indications for each treatment option shown by the dotted lines

Fig. 8.4 from Myers, KA, Sumner DS and Nicolaides AN. 1997: *Lower Limb Ischaemia*. London: Medorion.

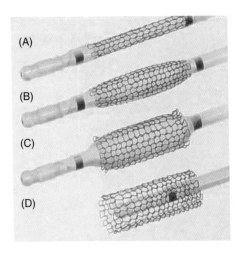

Fig. 8.11

A balloon-expandable stent

A: Balloon deflated and stent collapsed.

B: Balloon inflating.

C: Balloon fully inflated.

D: Stent fully expanded and balloon withdrawn.

and are encouraged that improvement is at least as likely as deterioration so that intervention may never be required.

Endovascular intervention

Many stenoses or occlusions can be effectively treated by balloon dilatation or stenting (Fig. 8.11).

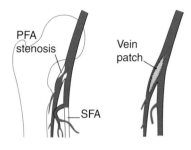

Fig. 8.12

Profunda endarterectomy and patch

Fig. 12.18 from Myers KA, Marshall RD and Freidin J. 1980: *Principles of Pathology*. Oxford: Blackwell. Reproduced with permission from Blackwell.

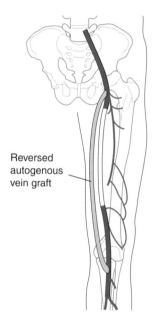

Fig. 8.13

Reversed autogenous femoropopliteal vein bypass graft

Fig. 5.9 from Myers KA, Marshall RD and Freidin J. 1980: *Principles of Pathology*. Oxford: Blackwell. Reproduced with permission from Blackwell.

Surgical endarterectomy

The atherosclerosis and inner layers of the media are peeled out, and the arterial incision is commonly patched with vein or synthetic material to widen the artery (Fig. 8.12).

Surgical bypass grafts

Autogenous vein is preferred for infrainguinal bypass grafting (Fig. 8.13). The vein can be reversed so that valves do not impede flow, or non-reversed *in situ* after breaking down valves and ligating tributaries.

The ipsilateral or contralateral long or short saphenous veins, or arm veins can be used. These may need to be scanned before operation to ensure that they are large enough and not thrombosed.

Synthetic grafts made from dacron or polytetrafluoroethylene (PTFE) are used for abdominal grafts (Fig. 8.14), or for infrainguinal grafts with an above-knee distal anastomosis, or when a suitable vein cannot be found. Composite grafts combining autogenous vein and a synthetic material can be used.

Amputation

Major below-knee or above-knee amputation is required in a small number of patients with critical ischaemia where there is no runoff artery to accept the distal anastomosis for a bypass graft, as shown by high-quality arteriography.

What the doctors need to know

Resting and post-exercise ankle/brachial pressure tests can determine:

- is arterial disease present?
- is disease unilateral or bilateral?
- what is the limiting factor for walking?
- how badly is walking limited?

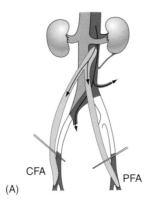

Fig. 8.14

Synthetic abdominal arterial bypass grafts

A: Aortobifemoral bypass.

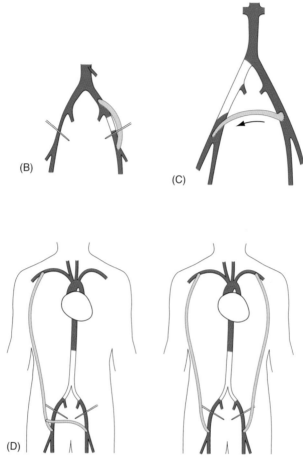

Fig. 8.14 (*continued*)

Synthetic abdominal arterial bypass grafts

B: Iliofemoral bypass

C: Femorofemoral bypass.

D: Unilateral or bilateral axillofemoral bypass.

A is taken from Fig. 13.10 from Queral L, in: Bergan JJ and Yao JS. 1979: *Surgery of the Aorta and its Body Branches*. New York: Grune and Stratton. Reproduced with permission.

A duplex scan is used to determine:

- the sites of disease
- whether there are multiple segments of disease
- whether each lesion is a stenosis or occlusion
- the severity of stenosis
- the length of each lesion.

CLINICAL ASPECTS: ANEURYSMS

Regional pathology

The distribution of aneurysms is different from that for occlusive disease (Fig. 8.15).

Ultrasound surveillance shows that abdominal aortic aneurysms (AAAs) expand on average by 3–4 mm per year. An AAA is unlikely to rupture until it reaches 5–5.5 cm diameter, and the corresponding diameter for iliac aneurysms is approximately 3 cm. As an AAA expands, laminated thrombus may accumulate on the aortic wall to maintain a normal flow channel.

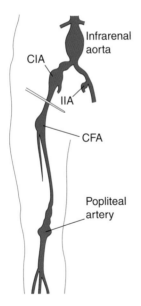

Fig. 8.15

Common sites for aneurysms in arteries to the lower limbs

The infrarenal abdominal aorta, CIA, CFA or popliteal artery.

Fig. 12.19 from Myers KA, Marshall RD and Freidin J. 1980: *Principles of Pathology*. Oxford: Blackwell. Reproduced with permission from Blackwell.

Clinical presentations

Asymptomatic AAAs are usually diagnosed by chance with:

- a pulsatile abdominal mass noticed by the patient
- clinical palpation, although many large AAAs are not detected in obese patients while a tortuous aorta can be misdiagnosed as AAA in a thin patient
- detection by a plain X-ray, showing calcification in the wall, ultrasound or computed tomography investigation for other abdominal or pelvic pathology.

Embolism of mural thrombus can cause the 'blue toe syndrome'. Retroperitoneal leakage or rupture will cause sudden severe abdominal or low back pain or shock.

Approximately 30 per cent of patients with AAAs also have popliteal aneurysms and vice versa.

CFA aneurysm may present with:

- a palpable mass in the groin
- rupture
- distal ischaemia from thrombosis.

Popliteal aneurysm may present with:

- a palpable popliteal fossa mass
- distal ischaemia from thrombosis
- calf muscle dysfunction and numbness from posterior tibial nerve compression
- calf swelling due to venous compression.

Treatment

AAA can be treated by open aortic bypass grafting (Fig. 8.16).

Many AAAs are now treated by endovascular aneurysm repair (EVAR) inserting a self-expanding endoluminal stent-graft through the CFAs (Fig. 8.17).

CFA and popliteal artery aneurysms are treated by synthetic or vein grafts or endovascular stent-grafts.

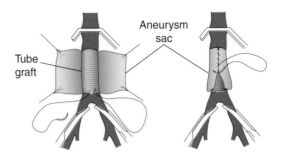

Fig. 8.16

Tube graft for AAA

A Dacron tube is anastomosed end-to-end to the infrarenal aorta and aortic bifurcation. The aneurysm sac is closed around the graft to separate it from overlying bowel.

Taken from Fig. 13.10 from Queral L, in: Bergan JJ and Yao JS. 1979: *Surgery of the Aorta and its Body Branches*. New York: Grune and Stratton. Reproduced with permission.

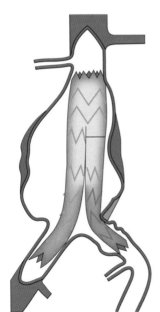

Fig. 8.17

Endovascular aneurysm repair

The stent-graft expands to make firm circumferential contact with a 'neck' of relatively normal aorta between the renal arteries and upper end of the AAA, as well as each CIA below the aneurysm.

What the doctors need to know

The choice between open or endoluminal grafting for AAA and **iliac aneurysms** depends on the anatomy. The aims are to:

- detect the presence of aneurysms
- measure the maximum diameter and length of the AAA
- show if there is mural thrombus and measure the residual lumen diameter
- record the length of normal aorta between the lowest renal artery and upper end of the AAA
- record where aneurysms finish in relation to the bifurcation or iliac arteries
- measure the diameters of the CFAs to ensure that they are large enough to be able to insert an endoluminal graft.

For **infrainguinal aneurysms**, the aims are to:

- detect the aneurysm
- determine its position and extent
- record its dimensions
- show if there is mural thrombus and measure the residual lumen diameter
- establish whether or not it is patent.

CLINICAL ASPECTS: NON-ATHEROSCLEROTIC DISEASES

Regional pathology

Pathology for several conditions is discussed on page 88 in Chapter 5. Other diseases are specific for arteries to the lower extremity.

- **Abdominal aortic coarctation.** A congenital aortic stricture can cause renovascular and lower limb ischaemia.
- **Aortic dissection.** Distal extension of dissection can occlude one or both common iliac arteries.
- **Takayasu's disease.** This frequently affects the abdominal aorta with occlusion of multiple visceral branches, or aortic and iliac artery stenoses.

- **Fibromuscular dysplasia.** This occasionally affects external iliac arteries with or without associated renal artery involvement.
- **Post-irradiation arteritis.** This usually follows irradiation for pelvic tumours such as carcinoma of the uterus, so as to cause common or external iliac stenosis or occlusion.
- **Arteriovenous fistulae.** These are abnormal communications from arteries to veins that may be congenital (multiple) or acquired (single) usually from iatrogenic trauma such as an arterial puncture.
- **Ergotism.** This affects larger iliac and femoral arteries rather than their smaller branches, with diffuse spasm or late occlusion.
- **Repetitive external iliac arterial trauma.** This can cause subintimal fibrosis in competition cyclists and other sportspersons. Characteristic findings are long stenoses from just beyond the EIA origin, with lengthening and tortuosity of the artery.
- **Buerger's disease.** This condition affects crural arteries with multiple occlusions and copious collaterals, usually with little or no involvement of arteries above the knees.
- **Cystic adventitial disease.** This causes popliteal artery stenosis that can progress to a short occlusion. Gelatinous material accumulates in the adventitia to cause smooth narrowing of the lumen (the scimitar sign), with normal proximal and distal arteries.
- **Tibial compartment syndrome.** This most often affects the anterior compartment and probably commences with impaired venous outflow leading to increased compartmental pressure and restricted arterial inflow. Clinical manifestations can range from aching to ischaemic necrosis.
- **Popliteal entrapment syndrome.** Entrapment results from an abnormal course of the popliteal artery in relation to the medial head of the gastrocnemius or other muscles (Fig. 8.18). Repeated trauma may lead to stenosis, post-stenotic aneurysm or thrombosis.
- **Persistent sciatic artery (PSA).** PSA arises from the IIA and passes through the greater sciatic notch:
  - It joins a normal popliteal artery in 90 per cent of cases but an incomplete form terminates at the back of the thigh in 10 per cent
  - The SFA is normal in 15 per cent but the remainder are hypoplastic or absent

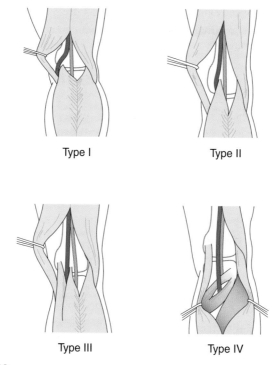

Type I

Type II

Type III

Type IV

Fig. 8.18

Popliteal artery entrapment

Entrapment by the medial head of gastrocnemius:

- type I (60–75 per cent): the artery is displaced medial to the muscle origin
- type II: the artery descends in a straight course medial to the muscle that arises more lateral than normal
- type III: the artery descends in a straight course medial to an accessory slip of muscle
- type IV: the artery is trapped by the popliteus, soleus or plantaris muscles or a fibrous band
- type V: there is no obvious anatomical abnormality.

Fig. 25.5 from Myers KA, Sumner DS and Nicolaides AN. 1997: *Lower Limb Ischaemia*. London: Medorion.

- Either the PSA or SFA provide a normal circulation in over 95 per cent and less than 5 per cent have incomplete arteries and ischaemia
- PSA is bilateral in 25 per cent

- About 50 per cent have an aneurysm just distal to the sciatic notch, particularly if the SFA is hypoplastic or absent.

CLINICAL ASPECTS: OTHER CONDITIONS

Arteriovenous graft for dialysis

A saphenous vein or synthetic bypass graft may be required to allow haemodialysis for chronic renal disease. This is commonly constructed between the common femoral artery and vein (Fig. 8.19). Ultrasound surveillance is used to ensure that the graft remains patent and functional (see page 250 in Chapter 11).

Mapping for free flaps

A free flap for plastic surgery to repair a tissue defect requires a suitable artery and veins to maintain its viability. A common donor site is a flap of skin and muscle from the lower abdominal wall based on the deep inferior epigastric vessels which arise from the EIA and pass to the external iliac vein on each side.

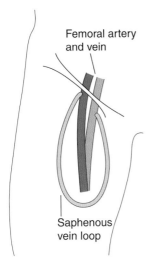

Femoral artery and vein

Saphenous vein loop

Fig. 8.19

Saphenous vein graft used for arteriovenous fistula to allow haemodialysis

Fig. 7.18 from Uldall R. 1988: *Renal Nursing*. Oxford: Blackwell. Reproduced with permission.

THE DUPLEX SCAN

An experienced sonographer can scan arteries from the aorta to the feet in both limbs in a reasonable time in more than 90 per cent of well-prepared patients. Ultrasound can accurately detect major artery disease with >90 per cent accuracy when compared with digital subtraction angiography (DSA). Distal disease may be less accurately assessed by ultrasound if there are multiple stenoses.

Box 8.3: Abbreviations
- PSV: peak systolic velocity
- EDV: end diastolic velocity
- V_2/V_1: ratio of PSV at and just proximal to a stenosis
- PSB: pansystolic spectral broadening

Normal findings

A high-resistance bi- or triphasic signal with no PSB and a range of PSVs, though no higher than 150 cm/s (Table 8.1).

Indications for scanning

Occlusive arterial disease

- Patients with equivocal symptoms or obscure diagnosis.

Table 8.1 Representative normal PSVs in lower limb arteries.

Artery	PSV (cm/s)
Aorta	75
CIA	110
EIA	110
CFA	90
Proximal SFA	90
Distal SFA	75
Popliteal	60
Crural	50

- Patients with clinical symptoms sufficient to warrant intervention using ultrasound to:
  - locate sites of serious disease to precisely plan for DSA
  - select patients for endovascular therapy without prior DSA.

The ultrasound scan can be equivocal and this then warrants a diagnostic DSA to:

- distinguish tight stenosis from occlusion
- assess the contribution from multiple stenoses
- detect and grade disease in crural arteries.

Opinion!

A good history and clinical examination are sufficient to assess many patients with typical symptoms and mild disability without the need to involve the vascular diagnostic service.

Surveillance after intervention for occlusive disease

Bypass grafts are subject to stenosis or occlusion (Fig. 8.20).

Graft stenosis may not cause recurrent symptoms and can be detected by ultrasound surveillance, although some grafts occlude without prior stenosis.

There is strong support for surveillance after autogenous vein grafting. The graft is monitored for:

- increased or reduced PSV in the graft, inflow and outflow arteries
- occlusion
- incorporation into surrounding tissues.

Traditional intervals for graft surveillance are:

- one month after operation
- three-monthly for one year
- bi-annually for the second year, then annually.

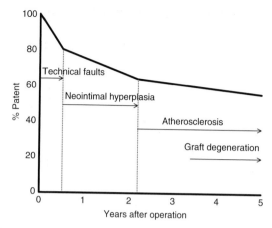

Fig. 8.20

Causes of graft failure

- First few weeks: technical faults.
- First 2 years: neointimal hyperplasia in the graft and at the anastomoses.
- After 2 years: atherosclerosis in the graft and inflow and outflow arteries.
- Later: graft degeneration.

Redrawn from Fig. 11.1 from van Reedt Dortland RWH, in: Chant ADB and Barros D'Sa AAB (eds). 1997: *Emergency Vascular Practice*. London: Hodder Arnold.

There is less support for routine surveillance after a synthetic graft or endovascular procedure but a positive finding can lead to correction of restenosis.

Aneurysms

Vascular ultrasound is a simple and reliable technique to assess AAA (Fig. 8.21) although other investigations are required if intervention is being considered.

Surveillance after EVAR

Integrity and a stable position are best shown by serial plain X-rays. The most important complication is 'endoleak' from within the graft back into the aneurysm sac and this is well seen with duplex scanning (Fig. 8.22).

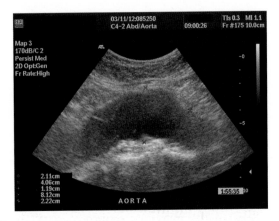

Fig. 8.21

B-mode of AAA in longitudinal showing diameter of the neck, maximum anteroposterior diameter, residual lumen diameter, aneurysm length and distal aortic diameter

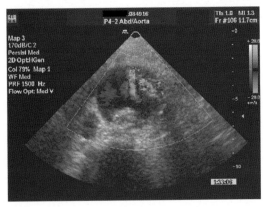

Fig. 8.22

Colour Doppler image of a type I endoleak from an endoluminal graft

Criteria for diagnosing occlusive disease

Lower limb arterial stenoses

These have been defined by comparing maximum PSV or V_2/V_1 ratio and waveform analysis with DSA. We use criteria derived by Cossman, Ellison and colleagues to assess lower limb arterial stenoses

Table 8.2 Criteria to define lower limb arterial stenoses.

Stenosis (%)	PSV (cm/s)	V_2/V_1 ratio
30–50	150–200	1.5–2
50–75	200–400	2–4
>75	>400	>4

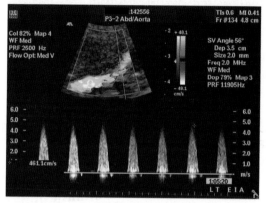

Fig. 8.23

Spectral analysis for an iliac artery with >75 per cent stenosis

(Table 8.2 and Fig. 8.23) (Cossman DV, Ellison JE, Wagner WH *et al. Journal of Vascular Surgery* 1989;**10**:522). There is no consensus as to whether PSV or V_2/V_1 is more accurate although V_2/V_1 may be preferred for multiple stenoses.

With increasing degrees of stenosis, the waveform shows progressive pansystolic broadening then post-stenotic turbulence. Severe stenosis may be associated with aliasing, monophasic or forward and reverse flow, and a shrill high-velocity signal.

Bypass graft stenosis

Most departments use V_2/V_1 to define significant graft stenosis with discriminant values reported from >1.5 to >3.0. A maximum PSV >350 cm/s or <45 cm/s also suggest imminent graft failure. Changes in the spectral waveform from tri- or biphasic to monophasic in the graft or inflow arteries indirectly predict graft stenosis. Duplex scanning is more reliable than ankle/brachial pressure indices which may not fall until stenosis is severe.

Lower limb arterial occlusion

Occlusion is diagnosed with confidence if there is:

● no colour Doppler or spectral signal in the occluded segment
● a high-resistance spectral signal above the segment
● a low-amplitude spectral signal below the segment
● a collateral leaving the artery at the top end
● a collateral re-entering the artery at the lower end.

Box 8.4: Plaque characteristics

Composition and echogenicity:
● homogeneous and hypoechoic
● heterogeneous and hyperechoic
● dense calcific with acoustic shadowing.

Surface:
● smooth and intact
● irregular
● ulcerated.

Aneurysms and EVAR

An AAA is defined as diameter >3 cm or diameter increased by more than 1.5 times normal.

Endoleaks after EVAR are classified as:

● type I: loss of contact between either end of graft and artery, or between modular components (Fig. 8.22)
● type II: flow into the sac from reversed flow in the inferior mesenteric or lumbar arteries or other aortic branches
● type III: flow through a tear in the fabric of the graft
● type IV: flow through interstices of the graft material.

PROTOCOLS FOR SCANNING

Follow principles for scanning described on pages 38 and 43 in Chapter 2.

Prepare the patient

Ask where pain occurs, when it comes on and what else interferes with walking. Take a history for past operations. Palpate lower limb pulses. Look for past incisions for surgery to help indicate the position of underlying bypass grafts. Scanning can be difficult if the patient is elderly, large, incapacitated or unable to move easily, has had an amputation or recent surgery, or has ulcers or gangrene.

Select the best transducer

- Scan abdominal arteries with a low-frequency curved array transducer.
- Use a phased array transducer if the patient is obese or gassy.
- Scan with a medium- to high-frequency linear array transducer for most infrainguinal arteries.
- Change to a curved array transducer for the SFA if the patient is large, has oedematous legs, at the adductor hiatus, or if the tibioperoneal trunk or peroneal artery are difficult to see because of heavy calcification or low flow.

Abdominal arteries

Opinion!

We consider that abdominal arteries should be scanned as part of the initial study for any patient being investigated for lower limb arterial disease. We do not consider that it is sufficient to infer whether abdominal arterial disease is present or absent by indirect assessment of CFA waveforms. Others disagree.

Position the patient and select a window

Scan with the patient lying supine and image the aorta from an anterior approach through the rectus abdominus muscles. Use techniques to avoid bowel gas described on page 51 in Chapter 3.

Scanning techniques for abdominal arteries

Some sonographers prefer to commence at the proximal abdominal aorta and work distally through the length of the iliac arteries.

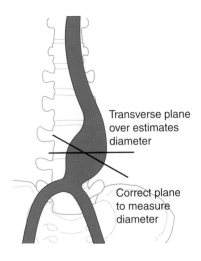

Transverse plane over estimates diameter

Correct plane to measure diameter

Fig. 8.24

Transverse diameter of AAA

Measure the true oblique diameter rather than the transverse plane which will overestimate the diameter if the aorta and AAA are tortuous.

Fig. 24.6 from Zwiebel WJ. 1992: *Introduction to Vascular Ultrasonography*. Philadelphia: WB Saunders. Reproduced with permission.

For the **aorta**:

- image with B-mode in transverse to measure the maximum infrarenal diameter
- image with B-mode to classify plaque type. Use colour Doppler in longitudinal to highlight aliasing. Use spectral Doppler to obtain PSVs proximal, at and distal to stenoses to classify severity, location and extent. Describe location of stenoses as suprarenal, proximal, mid or distal infrarenal aorta
- if there is an AAA, measure the true maximum transverse diameter in B-mode then change to longitudinal to measure the maximum anteroposterior diameter (Fig. 8.24)
- note mural thrombus and record the minimum residual lumen diameter. Use colour Doppler to help show the lumen if mural thrombus is echolucent
- measure diameters proximal and distal to the AAA. Note if dilatation extends suprarenally, involves the renal arteries or aortic bifurcation, and if tortuosity is present
- record the relation of the upper end of the AAA to the renal arteries and measure the length of the neck from the most distal renal artery.

For **iliac arteries:**

- use B-mode to classify plaque type, measure diameters, and note if they are tortuous or ectatic
- follow arteries in longitudinal with colour Doppler. Use spectral Doppler to obtain sample waveforms. Measure PSVs proximal, at and distal to sites of stenosis to assess severity, location and extent. Describe the stenosis location as origin, proximal, mid, distal or throughout.

> ## Note!
>
> Plaque and diameters must be classified with the colour turned off as this will increase spatial resolution.

Other sonographers prefer to start distally and work up to the aorta.

- Begin scanning at the inguinal ligament in longitudinal.
- Use colour Doppler to identify the distal EIA curving towards the transducer, and follow it proximally to the iliac bifurcation.
- Use colour Doppler to identify the IIA passing deep into the pelvis.
- Continue to scan the CIA to the abdominal aorta recognized by sudden change in diameter at the umbilicus.
- Take recordings as previously described.

Scanning techniques for surveillance after EVAR

The purpose is to detect an endoleak and classify its type, and to measure change in residual sac diameter. An endoleak is probably present if the residual lumen diameter increases with surveillance, and is not present if the AAA residual diameter has decreased. Surveillance may be discontinued if the sac disappears. A type I endoleak is present if colour and spectral Doppler show flow from the graft into the aneurysm sac. Reverse flow in an aortic branch with colour filling of the AAA residual lumen indicates a type II endoleak.

- Reduce colour scale to highlight low velocity flow.
- Use spectral Doppler to demonstrate flow direction in branches of the aorta.

● Use B-mode to measure diameters of the residual lumen of the AAA and limbs of the graft.

CFA, PFA and SFA

Position the patient and select a window

Examine the patient lying supine with the limb externally rotated. Turn the patient if necessary.

Tip!

Image quality may deteriorate as the SFA passes through the adductor hiatus in the lower third of thigh. Try straightening the leg and use an anterior approach through the vastus medialis muscle – the artery is further from the transducer but the image is improved.

Scanning techniques for the CFA, PFA and SFA

● Commence in longitudinal in the CFA just proximal to the inguinal ligament and progress down to the femoral bifurcation.
● Turn to transverse and use B-mode and colour Doppler to help identify the SFA and PFA origins.
● The PFA is lateral and deep to the SFA but it can be difficult to differentiate the two if either is occluded. The PFA has multiple branches.
● The femoral bifurcation is the landmark to measure the origin and length of a stenosis or occlusion in the SFA.
● Use colour Doppler to follow arteries in longitudinal.
● Take sample PSVs and record PSVs proximal to, at and distal to the sites of stenosis to classify severity, location and extent.
● If there is a CFA aneurysm, measure its maximum diameter and diameters in the normal artery just proximal and distal.

Tip!

Use the adjacent vein as a guide if the SFA is occluded, remembering that the vein is deep to the artery.

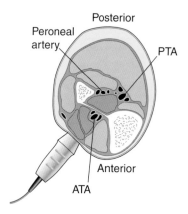

Fig. 8.25

Insonation of the ATA and accompanying veins

An anterolateral approach used particularly in the proximal leg as the ATA passes through the interosseous membrane.

Figs 4–6 from Zeigenbein RW, Myers KA, Matthews PG *et al. Phlebology* 1994;**9**:108–113. Reproduced with permission from Springer-Verlag, Heidelberg.

Popliteal and crural arteries

Position the patient and select a window

Turn the patient prone or on the side with the knee slightly flexed to view the popliteal artery, tibioperoneal trunk or peroneal artery. Scan for the anterior tibial artery through an anterolateral window (Fig. 8.25) with the patient supine and toes inverted. Scan for the posterior tibial and peroneal arteries from a medial approach (Fig. 8.26) with the patient supine and the leg flexed to drop the gastrocnemius muscles away. Considerable transducer pressure may be required. An alternative method to view crural arteries is to sit the patient with the foot on your knee to allow the calf muscles to drop away from the arteries and better fill veins as landmarks for the arteries (Fig. 10.19, page 21).

Scanning techniques for the popliteal artery

- Use B-mode and colour Doppler in transverse to identify the artery.
- Turn the transducer to show the artery in longitudinal.
- Use colour Doppler to determine arterial patency and the location of stenoses and occlusions.
- Use spectral Doppler to determine patency, particularly if calcified plaque causes shadowing to obscure colour Doppler. Record sample PSVs from at least one point in the popliteal artery .
- Record PSVs proximal to, at and distal to sites of stenosis and classify the severity, location and extent.

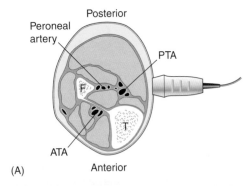

(A)

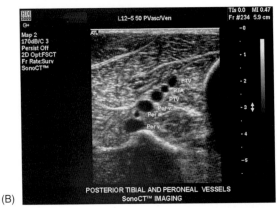

(B)

Fig. 8.26

Insonation of posterior tibial and peroneal vessels from a medial window in transverse

A: Orientation of probe. F: fibula; T: tibia.
B: B-mode image of arteries and veins.

Reproduced from Figs 4 and 5 from Zeigenbein RW, Myers KA, Matthews PG *et al. Phlebology* 1994;**9**:108–113, with the permission of the Royal Society of Medicine Press, London.

● Record PSVs proximal and distal to an occlusion and measure its location and length.
● Measure the position of the stenosis or occlusion in relation to the skin crease at the back of the knee or from the femoral bifurcation if a SFA stenosis is also present.

- If there is a popliteal aneurysm, use B-mode to measure its proximal, maximum and distal diameters. Note the presence of mural thrombus and residual diameter.

Scanning techniques for crural arteries

- Use B-mode and colour Doppler in transverse to identify the arteries.
- Turn the transducer to show the arteries in longitudinal.
- Veins are duplicated and lie next to each artery. Compress the foot or calf muscles to augment venous flow to help identify adjacent arteries.
- Use colour Doppler to follow each artery from its origin to the malleoli.
- Reduce the colour scale if necessary, as flow is often low compared with more proximal arteries.
- If none of the crural arteries are patent, scan the dorsalis pedis and medial plantar arteries for patency, as these can be used for the distal anastomoses for bypass grafts.
- Flow in crural arteries can be difficult to see if there is severe inflow disease.
- Describe the position of disease as at the origin, in the proximal, mid or distal artery, or throughout.
- Record sample PSVs from each distal crural artery.

Scanning techniques for bypass grafts

- Find the proximal anastomosis using B-mode and colour Doppler.
- Look for regions of inflow stenosis proximal to and at the proximal anastomosis. In B-mode, examine the proximal anastomosis for an aneurysm.
- Use colour Doppler in longitudinal to follow the graft to its distal anastomosis, looking for regions of stenosis.
- Take sample PSVs from the proximal, mid and distal graft and record PSVs proximal, at and distal to stenoses, to assess their severity, location, and extent in relation to the graft origin.

- Examine the distal anastomosis for aneurysm and stenosis.
- Examine distal outflow for stenosis and patency.
- Monitor the graft for incorporation into surrounding tissues or perigraft collection.

> ### Tip!
>
> When scanning grafts, remember that they have no branches and usually lie superficial to the native artery and vein. The anastomosis sites are dilated compared with the native artery and graft. The serrated walls of a Dacron graft and the venous sinuses of an autogenous vein graft are easily identified.

Scanning techniques for the popliteal entrapment syndrome

This is diagnosed by finding a normal appearance at rest changing to increased PSV or flow cessation with isometric active ankle plantarflexion or passive forced ankle dorsiflexion (Fig. 8.27). Duplex scanning can show some degree of popliteal artery and vein compression in normal subjects, particularly trained athletes with large muscles. Absence of the changes allows the diagnosis to be excluded.

Scanning techniques for arteriovenous fistulae

Look for:

- an 'arterialized venous signal' with spectral Doppler (Fig. 8.28)
- an increased pulse rate if connections are large
- varicose veins that may be pulsatile.

Abdominal wall flap mapping

The presence, length, diameter and branching of the deep inferior epigastric artery and veins on each side need to be documented before operation. The patency of anastomoses can be studied after operation.

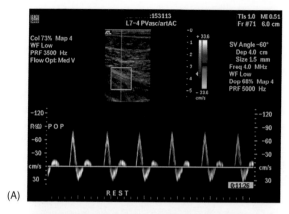

(A)

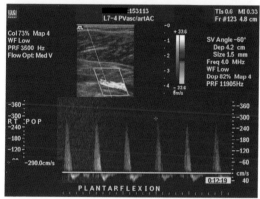

(B)

Fig. 8.27

Spectral Doppler signals with the popliteal entrapment syndrome in a popliteal artery

A: At rest.
B: During active isometric plantarflexion.

Reproduced from Fig. 6 from Zeigenbein RW, Myers KA, Matthews PG *et al. Phlebology* 1994;**9**:108–111, with the permission of the Royal Society of Medicine Press, London.

OTHER INVESTIGATIONS

The ankle/brachial pressure index (ABI)

This helps to establish whether disease is present.

ABI = ankle systolic pressure/brachial systolic pressure

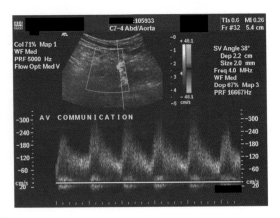

Fig. 8.28

Spectral Doppler signal from an arteriovenous fistula

Technique

- Lay the patient supine.
- Rest the patient for a consistent baseline.
- Apply sphygmomanometer cuffs to each arm over the brachial artery.
- Locate the brachial artery with CW Doppler.
- Inflate the cuff to 20–30 mmHg above the last audible pulse, and slowly deflate the cuff.
- Record the systolic pressure when flow resumes.
- Apply cuffs at each ankle and follow the same procedure for each dorsalis pedis artery and PTA. The peroneal artery can be used if it is the only patent artery to the ankle. Note the anatomy from Fig. 8.4.
- If available, use previous duplex studies to select which is the dominant crural artery.
- Use the highest ankle pressure (dorsalis pedis or posterior tibial) and highest of the two arm pressures to calculate the ABI.

Warning!

Cuffs should be applied snugly with the bladder over the artery to be compressed otherwise spuriously high pressures will be recorded.

Treadmill studies

The test measures walking distance and records systolic pressures at intervals after standard exercise on a treadmill. The walking distance measures disability and determines whether restriction agrees with the patient's history.

● Explain the procedure to the patient asking whether there are contraindications to exercise.
● Record resting ABIs. Leave the ankle cuffs on to allow for speedy assessment after exercise.
● Walk the patient on a motorized treadmill. A common protocol is to walk for up to 5 min at 2 km/h (33 m/min) on a 7 per cent slope. If the patient cannot cope, reduce the speed and note the settings.
● ECG monitoring can be performed.
● Immediately after exercise, measure brachial and ankle pressures from arteries that gave the highest readings before exercise, and then obtain ankle pressures every minute until pressures return to normal or for no more than 10 min.
● Record:
   ○ the time for onset of leg pain
   ○ where it occurs
   ○ the time when leg pain stops the patient from walking
   ○ any other reason for stopping.
      ○ dyspnoea,
      ○ angina,
      ○ joint pain,
      ○ fatigue or debility.
   ○ resting and serial post-exercise ABIs until recovery to the pre-exercise pressure.

Warning!

Do not exercise a patient with daily exertional angina or myocardial infarct less than 3 months before, unless a medical member of staff is present. Avoid performing exercise tests if the brachial systolic pressure is greater than 200 mmHg.

Clinical features

- If the resting ABI is reduced to <0.80 then occlusive disease is present. ABI >0.90 is considered normal.
- Differences in ABIs between the two limbs indicate whether disease is unilateral or bilateral, and which is more severely affected if disease is bilateral.
- If the resting ABI is normal but post-exercise ABIs fall, then early occlusive disease is present. If the post-exercise ABI remains normal then symptomatic occlusive disease can usually be excluded.
- Exercise will cause a decrease in ABI relative to the resting value – any apparent rise is due to technical error.
- There is debate as to the value of a post-exercise ABI if the resting ABI is already reduced.
- Observer variability is relatively high so that a decrease after exercise needs to be >0.15 to be significant.
- The test is invalid in some patients with heavily calcified crural arteries that are incompressible, particularly in diabetics.
- The ABI offers only an approximate estimate of disease severity.
- The ABI gives no information about where disease is located.
- Increases in ABIs accurately reflect a satisfactory response to treatment by bypass surgery or balloon dilatation.
- A falling ABI predicts a failing graft.

Segmental pressures

Segmental pressures can indicate the level of disease. Pressures can be obtained from three or more levels down the lower limb. A >20 mmHg pressure gradient between any two adjacent levels in the leg indicates significant disease in the intervening arterial segment. A >20 mmHg difference between sides at the same level indicates occlusive disease on the side with the lower pressure.

> ## Warning!
>
> Do not inflate a cuff over a bypass graft or stent for fear of causing it to occlude. Inform the patient that cuff inflation can cause discomfort.

Indices can also be calculated from thigh, calf or toe pressures.

Thigh pressures are normally recorded as higher than ankle or arm pressures (normal thigh/brachial index = 1.10–1.20). Wider cuffs are required.

Toe pressures are measured by infrared photoplethysmography with a 1.2 cm width cuff placed around the first toe. Toe pressures are normally recorded as lower than ankle or arm pressures (normal toe/brachial index = 0.80–0.90).

Arterial waveforms

An abnormal CW tracing with dampening of the waveform in the CFA at rest or after exercise indicates that there is proximal disease. However, a normal tracing does not exclude disease. Mathematical indices are now rarely used. CW waveforms may also be assessed at the popliteal artery, PTA and ATA.

Box 8.5: Ultrasound images to record

For the aorta and each side:
- occlusive disease and graft surveillance:
  - sample spectral traces in longitudinal for each artery listed in Box 8.1
  - sample spectral traces in the artery above and below a bypass graft and in the proximal, mid and distal graft
  - spectral traces proximal to and at each stenosis, noting their location and extent
  - spectral traces proximal and distal to occlusions, noting their location and extent.
  - B-mode of plaques in longitudinal
- aneurysms:
  - B-mode of the length of aneurysm in longitudinal
  - B-mode of maximum transverse and anteroposterior diameters of the aneurysm
  - B-mode of mural thrombus and residual lumen diameter of aneurysm
  - B-mode of the proximal and distal diameters of adjacent normal artery

---

- EVAR surveillance:
  - B-mode for maximum residual AAA and iliac artery diameters in transverse and longitudinal
  - colour Doppler for endoleaks at all levels
- further abnormalities such as non-atherosclerotic diseases indicating their location and extent.

9

VENOUS THROMBOSIS IN THE LOWER LIMBS

Ultrasound scanning is the investigation most often used to determine the presence, site and extent of thrombus in deep or superficial veins. The D-dimer pathology test has a high negative predictive value and can be used for screening. Occasionally, patients require venography to demonstrate iliac or inferior vena caval thrombosis. Computed tomographic and magnetic resonance angiography have a place in detecting intra-abdominal and pelvic thrombosis. Most departments have abandoned other indirect investigations.

ANATOMY

Box 9.1: Veins scanned for reporting*
- Common femoral vein: CFV
- Profunda femoris vein: PFV
- Femoral vein (previously superficial femoral vein): FV
- Popliteal vein
- Posterior tibial veins: PTV
- Peroneal veins
- Great saphenous vein (previously greater, long, internal): GSV
- Small saphenous vein (previously lesser, short, external): SSV
- Gastrocnemius veins and soleal sinuses

Other veins discussed
- Inferior vena cava: IVC
- Saphenofemoral junction: SFj
- Saphenopopliteal junction: SPj
- Anterior tibial veins: ATV

* The terminology used is in accordance with recommendations referred to in Chapter 10 (see Box 10.1, page 200).

Axial deep veins that may be affected by thrombosis are shown in Figs 9.1–9.3 and superficial veins in the lower limbs are described in Chapter 10.

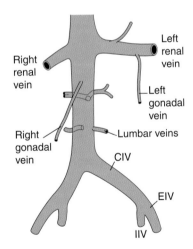

Fig. 9.1

The infrarenal IVC and iliac veins

- The IVC is to the right of the aorta.
- Each CIV is to the right of the corresponding artery.
- The left CIV is crossed by the right common iliac artery.
- The right gonadal (testicular or ovarian) vein joins the IVC.
- The left gonadal vein joins the left renal vein – it may be duplicated.

EIV: external iliac vein; IIV: internal iliac vein.

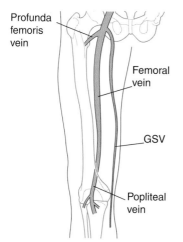

Profunda femoris vein

Femoral vein

GSV

Popliteal vein

Fig. 9.2

The femoral and popliteal veins

- The veins wind around the corresponding arteries.
- They are larger than the arteries.
- The FV and popliteal veins are duplicated in 10 per cent of limbs.

Figure kindly supplied by personal communication from Trevor Beckwith, Wagga Wagga, Australia, 1996.

Fig. 9.3

Crural veins, gastrocnemius veins and soleal sinuses

- The PTVs, ATVs and peroneal veins follow their corresponding arteries.
- They are usually duplicated.
- The ATV passes through the interosseous membrane.
- The gastrocnemius veins and soleal sinuses are paired and pass to the medial and lateral parts of the corresponding muscles.

Figure kindly supplied by personal communication from Trevor Beckwith, Wagga Wagga, Australia, 1996.

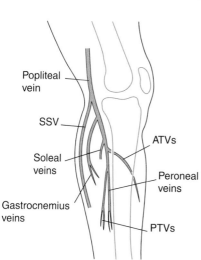

Popliteal vein

SSV

Soleal veins

Gastrocnemius veins

ATVs

Peroneal veins

PTVs

CLINICAL ASPECTS

Regional pathology, clinical presentations and treatment

Venous thrombosis can cause superficial thrombophlebitis or deep vein thrombosis (DVT), and these can lead to pulmonary embolism (PE). The pathology and risk factors for DVT are discussed on page 79 in Chapter 5.

Superficial thrombophlebitis

Thrombosis most often involves the GSV, SSV or major tributaries. The onset is acute and there is considerable surrounding inflammation often incorrectly thought to represent infection. The affected vein is painful, red, hot, easily palpable and tender. Thrombus propagates through the saphenous junctions or perforators to deep veins in approximately 10 per cent of limbs, and some 10 per cent of these detach to cause PE. Superficial thrombophlebitis is best treated by a compression bandage and analgesics, or by saphenous vein ligation. Anticoagulation is not required and antibiotics are inappropriate.

Deep vein thrombosis

DVT is considerably more common in the lower than upper limbs. Most DVTs commence in below-knee veins and approximately 10 per cent propagate to above-knee veins. If a scan is positive for DVT then some 30 per cent are bilateral. If the initial scan clearly excludes DVT, conversion to a positive scan is extremely unlikely.

A large proportion of patients with DVT have no symptoms or signs. The first presentation may be with PE or the condition may be unrecognized until the post-thrombotic syndrome develops many years later (see page 92, Chapter 5). Approximately 50 per cent of patients develop symptoms due to the post-thrombotic syndrome within 10 years after a major DVT.

If DVT becomes symptomatic then clinical features include acute pain, swelling, calf tenderness and a moderately raised temperature. Extensive iliofemoral thrombosis can reduce the circulation sufficiently to threaten viability of the leg and this is termed **phlegmasia cerulea dolens**. Many patients studied for pain or swelling in the leg do not have a DVT, but more than 50 per cent of these have another condition that can be diagnosed by ultrasound.

DVT is now usually treated in the outpatient department with compression bandaging and anticoagulation with low molecular weight heparin injections initially and oral warfarin for 3–6 months. Occasionally, patients with iliofemoral thrombosis are treated by thrombolysis or surgical thrombectomy.

Pulmonary embolism

Thrombus may break away from veins to pass through the right atrium and ventricle to the pulmonary arteries as a PE. Approximately 10–20 per cent of lower limbs with DVT develop PE, which is most likely in the early stages of thrombosis when the clot is less adherent.

A patent foramen ovale is present in approximately 30 per cent of the population and it is possible for an embolus to pass through from the right to left atrium to the arterial circulation, frequently moving to the brain causing stroke; this is **paradoxical embolism.**

According to the size of the embolus, presentation may be silent and only detected by investigations to give four different forms of presentation: symptomatic without compromising the circulation, catastrophic causing cardiac shock, or fatal. Symptoms of PE include deep chest pain, pleuritic pain and dyspnoea. For patients with possible PE, ultrasound is positive for DVT in approximately 40 per cent if an isotope lung scan is clearly positive, 15 per cent if the lung scan is equivocal and 10 per cent if the lung scan is normal.

PE is treated by anticoagulation in hospital. Recurring PE despite adequate anticoagulation is an indication to place an IVC filter. Occasionally, patients with severe circulatory impairment require thrombolysis or pulmonary embolectomy.

Differential diagnosis of deep vein thrombosis

In approximate order of frequency:

- cellulitis
- torn calf muscle
- ruptured Baker's cyst
- subfascial haematoma
- ruptured plantaris muscle
- prolonged limb dependency
- lymphoedema
- lymphangitis
- nerve entrapment.

What the doctors need to know

- **Is there venous thrombosis?** Many patients are asymptomatic and many symptomatic patients have other conditions.
- **Is there thrombus in superficial veins and how close is it to the saphenous junction?** GSV thrombophlebitis extending to the SFj may require urgent surgery to ligate the junction to prevent PE.
- **Is there projection of thrombus into the deep vein?** This observation markedly increases the risk of PE.
- **Is there thrombus in deep veins and if so where?** This is almost always an urgent indication to commence early treatment to reduce the risk of complications.
- **Is the process unilateral or bilateral?** This does not affect immediate treatment but is of value to assess the early risk of PE and long-term prognosis for the post-thrombotic syndrome.
- **Do serial studies show that a DVT is propagating?** If so, then the efficacy of treatment may need to be reviewed.
- **Do serial studies show that the vein is recanalizing or remaining occluded?** This can influence the duration for anticoagulation.

Warning!

If there is any doubt about the diagnosis, call the supervising doctor to check the findings. The sonographer or supervising doctor should ring the referring doctor immediately if DVT or floating thrombus in a proximal saphenous vein are detected. Do not send the patient home before determining appropriate management. This is a very important scan with the onus on the sonographer to be sure before declaring the study to be normal.

THE DUPLEX SCAN

Studies that compare ultrasound scanning with venography show that the sensitivity for ultrasound is >95 per cent for above-knee thrombosis, and >85 per cent for below-knee thrombosis for scans where adequate imaging is obtained.

Characteristics of normal veins

Ultrasound features characteristic for normal veins:

- compressible with transducer pressure (Fig. 9.4)
- thin-walled
- larger than the corresponding artery
- smooth interior lumen
- echo-free lumen
- augment with distal compression causing full colour filling of the lumen
- show phasic flow with respiration and cessation of flow with the Valsalva manoeuvre in upper thigh veins
- increase of the CFV diameter by 15–20 per cent with the Valsalva manoeuvre.

Indications for scanning

Patients may be referred with symptoms or signs suggesting superficial thrombophlebitis, DVT or PE. Alternatively, asymptomatic patients may be referred if considered to be at high risk due to recent surgery,

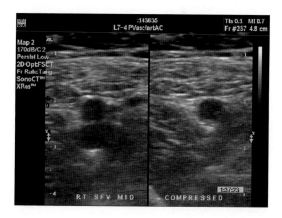

Fig. 9.4

B-mode appearance of a normal CFV prior to compression (left) and after transducer compression (right)

prolonged bed rest, lower limb trauma or known thrombophilia. The approximate yield is:

- leg pain or swelling suspected due to DVT: 30 per cent
- DVT as a suspected source of PE: 20 per cent
- asymptomatic patients referred to exclude DVT: 15 per cent.

Box 9.2: Patient surveillance

There is no agreement as to how to follow the patient after a DVT is confirmed. We perform weekly scans until the thrombus is recanalized. This may be used to determine the duration for anticoagulation.

Criteria for diagnosing thrombosis
Direct evidence for thrombosis

- **Inability to compress the vein.** Thrombus prevents the vein walls from coming together with compression. The vein can be partially compressed with a partially occlusive thrombus but is incompressible with a fully occlusive thrombus (Fig. 9.5).

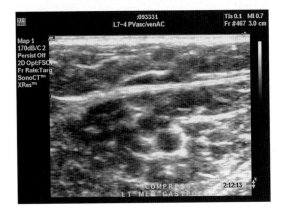

Fig. 9.5

Incompressible thrombus in medial gastrocnemius veins

- **Intraluminal clot.** A fresh clot is echolucent while an old thrombus is increasingly echogenic. This feature is highly dependent on image quality and instrument settings.
- **Absent flow in the vein.** There is no flow with occlusive thrombosis and only peripheral flow around a central non-occlusive thrombus (Fig. 9.6). This is an important indicator for iliac DVT where it is often not possible to test for compressibility.
- **Diameter of the vein.** The diameter increases from the bulk of thrombus in the acute phase (Fig. 9.7) and then gradually shrinks to become smaller than normal in the chronic phase.
- **Thickening of the vein wall.** The wall thickness gradually increases with time.

Indirect evidence for thrombus

- **Loss of phasic flow** with respiration or little or no response to the Valsalva manoeuvre in the CFV suggests obstruction proximal to the examination site (Fig. 5.11, page 95). However, normal spectral Doppler cannot exclude DVT since there may be only partial thrombosis in the abdominal veins. Of these criteria, this requires the most experience.
- **Loss of change of diameter** in the CFV with the Valsalva manoeuvre suggests proximal occlusive thrombosis.

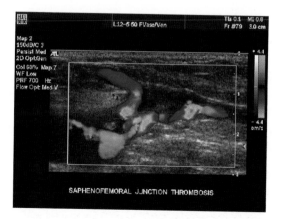

Fig. 9.6

Colour Doppler showing flow around an incompletely occlusive thrombus at the saphenofemoral junction

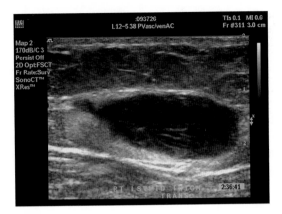

Fig. 9.7

Superficial thrombophlebitis showing marked distension of the greater saphenous vein

● **Minimal augmentation** of flow after calf compression suggests occlusion between the examination and augmentation sites.
● **Increased flow in superficial veins** because they are acting as collaterals.
● **Deep collaterals.**

Note!

Deep veins always accompany their corresponding arteries and this helps to correctly identify deep veins rather than collaterals, particularly if chronic thrombosis has caused a vein to atrophy.

Ultrasound findings relating to the age of thrombus

There are several characteristic ultrasound features.

Acute thrombosis

● loss of compressibility
● thrombus with low echogenicity
● increased vein diameter

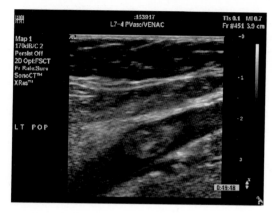

Fig. 9.8

'Free-floating' thrombus in the popliteal vein

- free-floating thrombus (Fig. 9.8)
- no flow on distal augmentation or the Valsalva manoeuvre.

Subacute thrombosis

- lost or partial compressibility
- increased thrombus echogenicity
- reduced vein diameter
- thrombus adherent to wall
- recanalization.

Chronic thrombosis

- partial compressibility
- moderate to marked thrombus echogenicity
- reduced vein diameter – it may be atrophied
- collateral flow in the region
- recanalization
- thick vein wall.

PROTOCOLS FOR SCANNING

Follow general principles for venous scanning described on page 40 in Chapter 2.

> ## Warning!
>
> With repeated tests for surveillance after DVT, ensure that levels for the extent of thrombus for each test are taken from the same bone, surface or confluence landmarks.

Prepare the patient

Pain is often felt at the site of thrombosis. Femoropopliteal DVT may result in calf oedema while iliac thrombosis often causes thigh and calf oedema. The referring doctor may indicate whether iliac veins are to be scanned, but if not then a history and examination of pain or swelling in the thigh, recent pregnancy or past iliac DVT should persuade you to include iliac veins in the study. The ultrasound scan can be difficult if the patient is obese. Bowel gas can obscure abdominal scanning and fasting the patient prior to the examination helps to give a better view (see page 37 in Chapter 2). Warn the patient that compression is part of the test and can be uncomfortable or painful.

Select the best transducer

Use a medium- to high-frequency linear array transducer to examine infrainguinal veins. Change to a lower frequency curved array transducer to examine iliac veins or the IVC, or to give better penetration if the thigh or calf is very oedematous. Oedema in the limb is confined to tissues superficial to the deep fascia, and this can obscure superficial veins or increase the depth for scanning deep veins.

Veins above knee: CFV, SFj and femoral confluence
Position the patient and select a window

Scan on a tilt table with the patient in reverse Trendelenburg at 30°. Lay the patient comfortably supine with the affected leg externally rotated and contralateral hip raised and slightly supported with a foam pad. The leg should be non-weight-bearing. Pain from DVT can be intense, making it difficult to scan, and you may have to alter the position to access veins with the least discomfort.

Scanning techniques for the CFV, SFj and femoral confluence

- Use B-mode in transverse to scan in the inguinal region. Identify the CFV medial to the corresponding artery and identify the SFj. Use spectral Doppler in longitudinal to help distinguish the CFV from the artery.

- Centre the CFV on the image in transverse and gently press to see if the CFV can be fully compressed by the transducer. Use B-mode and colour Doppler to see if the vein is fully or partially occluded and whether thrombus is 'free floating'.

- Assess the CFV with colour and spectral Doppler in longitudinal. Look for phasicity with normal respiration and cessation of flow with the Valsalva manoeuvre to show that proximal veins are patent. Colour should fill the lumen of the vessel with distal augmentation.

- Slowly move distally to identify the SFj and confluence of the SFV and PFV. Test for compressibility and normal Doppler characteristics.

- If present, note how near the thrombus is to a selected landmark and measure the thrombus length.

- Enlarged lymph nodes in the groin can be confused with a mass of thrombus, but they can be distinguished since lymph nodes are closed ended.

Note!

Do not compress the vein any more than necessary if there has been recent thrombosis for fear of detaching thrombus to cause PE.

SFV and GSV above the knee

Position the patient and select a window

Start with the patient on the tilt table as previously described. Scanning at the adductor hiatus can be difficult in some limbs and a posterior view may give a better image.

> **Tip!**
>
> It can be difficult to compress the distal FV when imaging through the anteromedial window. If so, place your free hand behind the thigh and push the limb into the transducer rather than trying to compress the vein through the adductor muscle.

Scanning techniques for the SFV

- Use B-mode to identify the origin of the SFV in transverse, just as for the CFV, and again check for compressibility.
- Continue down the SFV to the knee. Move the transducer down the medial thigh and compress every 1–2 cm.
- When you reach the adductor hiatus, start working posteriorly and then return to a more anterior approach in the distal thigh.
- Use colour Doppler at 1–2 cm intervals to show vein patency by augmentation after calf or distal thigh compression.
- If it is not certain that thrombus is present with B-mode, use spectral analysis to confirm that there is no flow.
- If thrombus is present, measure its extent from the knee crease or inguinal ligament.

> **Note!**
>
> Remember that the FV and popliteal vein may be duplicated and both veins need to be assessed. Adjacent arteries and nerves can be confused with veins during ultrasound examinations.

Scanning techniques for the above-knee GSV

- Use B-mode in transverse to check for compressibility of the GSV. Then use colour Doppler to check for full colour filling with distal augmentation.
- If the vein is incompressible, follow the thrombus through the length of the GSV and major tributaries to the knee crease.
- If thrombus is identified, measure its location from the SFj or knee crease.

> ## Warning!
>
> Initially, do not press too hard since the normal vein collapses very easily making it difficult to find.

Veins in the popliteal fossa

Position the patient and select a window

In reverse Trendelenburg, place the patient prone or on the side with the knee flexed. Alternatively, scan with the patient seated on the side of the bed with the leg dependent, or standing facing away with the weight on the other leg.

Scanning techniques for veins in the popliteal fossa

- Recommence scanning from behind the knee in transverse to identify the single or paired popliteal vein which is usually superficial to the popliteal artery.
- Assess the vein for compressibility and patency as far proximal as possible. Extra force may be needed to compress the vein.
- As you reach the mid-popliteal vein, you will see several tributaries including the SSV and gastrocnemius veins.
- The gastrocnemius and soleal veins are common sites for thrombosis. They are always paired and often contain stagnant blood that may resemble fresh thrombus.
- Examine the paired medial and lateral gastrocnemius veins from their confluence with the popliteal vein to as far down into the gastrocnemius muscles as possible.
- Examine the soleal sinuses which are situated lower and deeper in the calf than the gastrocnemius veins. They are frequently only visible if distended with thrombus.
- View the SSV in this region and test for compressibility and patency down the posterior calf.
- Before leaving the popliteal fossa, check for the presence and integrity of a Baker's cyst (Fig. 9.9).

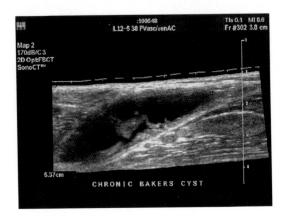

Fig. 9.9
A Baker's cyst in the popliteal fossa

Crural veins and distal GSV

Position the patient and select a window

Scan with the patient seated on the side of the bed with the leg dependent on the sonographer's knee (Fig. 10.19, page 221). Alternatively, scan with the patient supine and tilted into reverse Trendelenburg with the limb externally rotated. From the popliteal fossa, continue scanning from behind until the popliteal vein divides. Then scan from the medial or posteromedial aspect for the PTV and peroneal veins (see page 221 in Chapter 10). The peroneal veins can also be seen through a posterior or anterolateral window. We consider that ATV thrombosis is so rare that it is not worth scanning these veins.

Scanning techniques for crural veins and the distal GSV

- Assess the GSV and tributaries below the knee and measure the thrombus from the medial malleolus or knee crease.
- Assess the crural veins with calf muscle compression. Lack of augmentation indicates probable femoropopliteal or crural vein obstruction.
- Continue down the calf to the ankle in transverse, compressing each crural vein at regular intervals.
- Assess flow characteristics by augmenting the distal calf or foot. Spontaneous flow is not seen in crural veins.

● Use colour Doppler to check for patency, although this will not always exclude partial thrombosis.

IVC and iliac veins

The examination should extend to assess these veins in patients with thrombosis extending to the inguinal ligament or if flow patterns in the CFV suggest proximal occlusion. If iliac veins need to be examined then it is best to do this last as you will need to change to the lower frequency curved or phased array transducer for deeper penetration.

● It is difficult to compress abdominal veins.
● Use colour Doppler to follow iliac veins to the IVC. Loss of colour flow may suggest occlusive thrombus.
● Sample a Doppler signal from the vein to confirm loss of flow. If flow is seen throughout the iliac veins and IVC then the veins are patent although they could still be partially thrombosed.

Pitfalls and limitations!

● It can be difficult to compress normal veins at deep sites or if there is pain from the thrombus.
● Flow is present through partially thrombosed veins.
● The age of the thrombus is difficult to define.

Box 9.3: Ultrasound images to record

● Use B-mode to assess veins listed in Box 9.1. Use dual image to demonstrate a non-compressed and compressed vein beside each other.
● If thrombus is detected, use B-mode in transverse and longitudinal to show its location and extent in relation to landmarks.
● Sample Doppler traces in longitudinal for flow in the CFV with normal respiration and Valsalva.
● Sample colour images during augmentation for all veins listed.
● Other pathology such as lymphoedema or a Baker's cyst.

10

CHRONIC VENOUS DISEASE IN THE LOWER LIMBS

Ultrasound detects connections between deep and superficial veins, reflux in deep, superficial and perforator veins, or venous obstruction. Continuous-wave Doppler supplements clinical assessment but duplex scanning is required to define anatomy. Venography is occasionally performed prior to surgery. Air plethysmography is favoured for physiological assessment, but other plethysmographic techniques are now rarely used. This chapter includes findings from our experience with 7000 chronic venous duplex scans.

ANATOMY

Box 10.1: Veins scanned for reporting*

- Great saphenous vein (previously greater, long, internal): GSV
- Small saphenous vein (previously lesser, short, external): SSV
- Anterior and posterior accessory saphenous veins: AASV and PASV
- Anterior and posterior thigh circumflex veins (previously anterior and posterior thigh veins) ATCV and PTCV

- Thigh extension of SSV: TE
- Vein of Giacomini
- Saphenofemoral junction: SFj
- Saphenopopliteal junction: SPj
- Gastrocnemius and soleal veins
- Thigh and calf perforators
- Superficial tributaries
- Common femoral vein: CFV
- Profunda femoris vein: PFV
- Femoral vein (previously superficial femoral vein): FV
- Popliteal vein
- Posterior tibial veins: PTV
- Peroneal veins

Other veins discussed
- Inferior vena cava: IVC
- Common, internal and external iliac veins: CIV, IIV, EIV
- Ovarian veins
- Anterior tibial veins: ATV

*The terminology is in accordance with recommendations from a consensus statement on behalf of the International Union of Phlebology, International Federations of Associations of Anatomists, and Federative International Committee on Anatomical Terminology: *Journal of Vascular Surgery* 2002;**36**:416–422. Each service has its own terminology which must be made clear if abbreviations are used.

Ultrasound for chronic venous disease particularly studies the GSV and AASV (Figs 10.1–10.4), SSV (Figs 10.5–10.6, page 204), TE and vein of Giacomini (Fig. 10.7, page 205; Carlo Giacomini (1840–1898), Professor of Anatomy at University of Turin, Italy), perforators (Fig. 10.8, page 205) and deep veins (see page 182 in Chapter 9).

CLINICAL ASPECTS

Regional pathology

Primary venous disease

- **Varicose veins**: large veins that bulge above the skin surface, usually affecting saphenous vein tributaries.

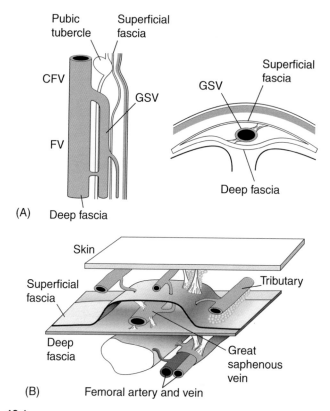

Fig. 10.1

GSV: relation to superficial fascia

- The SFj position is constant, just lateral to the pubic tubercle.
- The GSV lies within a superficial fascial compartment, the 'saphenous eye'.
- All tributaries including the ATCV and PTCV become superficial to this fascia.

A: Redrawn from Fig. 1 from Caggiati A. *Phlebology* 1997;**12**:107–111, with the permission of the Royal Society of Medicine Press, London.
B: Reprinted from Fig.1, Caggiati A, Bergan A, Gloviczki P *et al.*
Nomenclature of the veins of the lower limbs: an international interdisciplinary consensus statement. *Journal of Vascular Surgery* © 2002;**36**:416–422, with permission from the Society for Vascular Surgery.

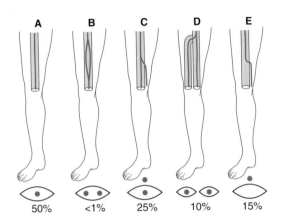

Fig. 10.2

GSV: variations in the distal thigh and proximal calf

● GSV is present continuously to ankle.

A: No major tributaries.
B: One or two major tributaries below the knee.
C: A major tributary that joins above the knee.

● GSV is not present continuously at the knee.

D: Absence of considerable length above and below the knee.
E: Absence of short length above and below the knee.

Redrawn from Fig. 2 from Ricci S. *Phlebology* 1999;**14**:59–64, with the permission of the Royal Society of Medicine Press, London.

● **Reticular veins:** smaller blue veins that do not protrude.
● **Telangiectases:** tiny, short unconnected or spidery branching vessels.

Reflux in the GSV
Duplex scanning shows variations in patterns of GSV reflux (Fig. 10.9, page 206). The frequencies are different in males and females.

Reflux in the SSV
Duplex scanning shows variations in patterns of SSV reflux (Fig. 10.10, page 207). The frequencies are the same for both sexes.

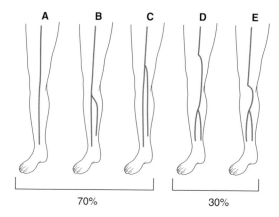

Fig. 10.3

GSV and AASV: variations in the thigh

A: Single GSV in its fascial compartment.
B: True duplication of the GSV in the one fascial compartment – very uncommon.
C: Single GSV and associated major superficial tributaries.
D: GSV and AASV each in separate fascial compartments.
E: Short length of GSV that then emerges to a superficial layer.

Redrawn from Fig. 1 from Ricci S. *Phlebology* 2002;**16**:111–116, with the permission of the Royal Society of Medicine Press, London.

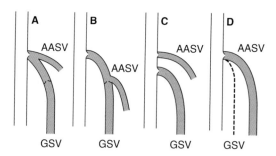

Fig. 10.4

Variations in origin of the AASV

A: Common junction with GSV.
B: Origin from GSV below SFj.
C: Origin from CFV above SFj.
D: Origin from SFj as principal vein with hypoplastic or absent GSV.

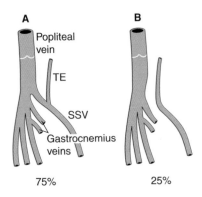

Fig. 10.5

SSV: variations in its termination

The TE is present in 95 per cent of limbs and is the continuation of the SSV.

A: The SSV may join the popliteal vein or deep veins at a higher level.

B: There may be no connection to deep veins.

- The SSV may be in the midline or medial or lateral to the midline.
- The gastrocnemius veins may join the popliteal vein, upper SSV, or confluence at the SPj.
- The soleal veins join the popliteal vein.

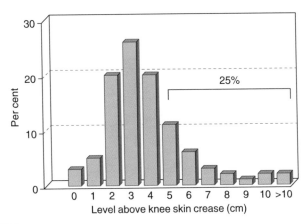

Fig. 10.6

SSV: level of SPj from our studies

- The level is variable.
- It is most often 2–4 cm above the knee crease.
- 25 per cent are higher than this level.
- The junction is rarely below the knee crease.

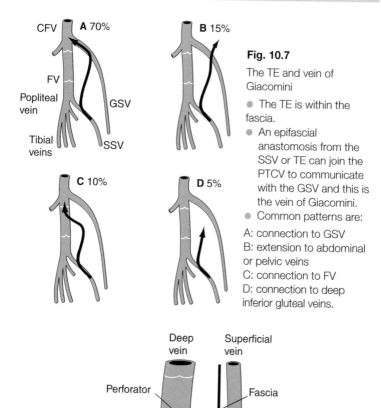

Fig. 10.7

The TE and vein of Giacomini

- The TE is within the fascia.
- An epifascial anastomosis from the SSV or TE can join the PTCV to communicate with the GSV and this is the vein of Giacomini.
- Common patterns are:

A: connection to GSV
B: extension to abdominal or pelvic veins
C: connection to FV
D: connection to deep inferior gluteal veins.

Fig. 10.8

Perforators

- They pass through the deep fascia to connect deep and superficial veins.
- A valve normally directs flow from superficial to deep.
- Thigh perforators usually pass from the GSV to the FV.
- Calf perforators can pass from the GSV, SSV or major tributaries to crural veins or to calf muscle venous plexuses.
- In order of frequency, calf perforators are on the medial, posterior, lateral or anterior aspects.

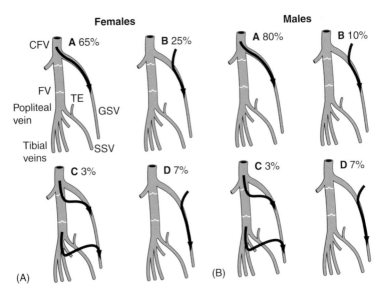

Fig. 10.9

Connections to the GSV territory with primary varicose veins from our studies

A: Females.
B: Males.

- The sources for reflux are:

1: SFj
2: low pelvic or abdominal veins
3: perforators
4: unknown sources.

- The destinations for reflux are the GSV, ATCV, PTCV or other tributaries.

Reflux in the TE or vein of Giacomini

Flow may be in either direction (Fig. 10.11).

Recurrent varicose veins

At least 30 per cent of patients develop recurrent varicose veins within 3–5 years after surgery. There are three reasons why varicose veins may appear after previous treatment:

- persistent **residual veins** in the territory due to failure to interrupt refluxing deep to superficial connections

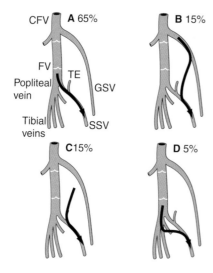

Fig. 10.10

Connections to SSV territory with primary varicose veins from our studies

- The sources for reflux are:

A: SPj

B: GSV tributaries

C: TE

D: popliteal perforators.

- The destinations of reflux are the SSV, TE, gastrocnemius veins or tributaries.

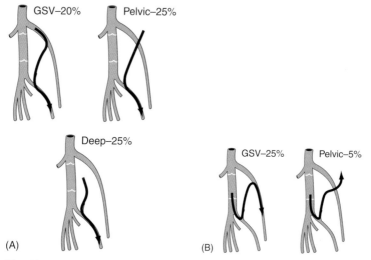

Fig. 10.11

Flow in the TE and vein of Giacomini

A: Flow may pass downwards into the SSV from the GSV, pelvic tributaries or deeper veins.

Flow may pass upwards into the GSV or pelvic veins from the SSV.

- true **recurrence** in the venous territory that was previously treated
- development of **new varicose veins** in a territory other than that previously treated.

Patterns of reflux are even more complex than for untreated varicose veins. Recurrence after surgery for GSV reflux affects the GSV territory in two-thirds or new disease with SSV or perforator reflux in one-third. Recurrence in the GSV territory may be due to reconnection at the SFj but many have connections at other sites (Fig. 10.12). Frequently, there are multiple deep to superficial connections. Similar considerations apply to the SPj after SSV surgery where veins from the popliteal fossa connect to the SSV or calf tributaries.

Deep venous disease

Deep venous reflux may involve the full length of the limb or isolated venous segments. Brief reverse flow over a short deep segment with no superficial reflux is assumed to be normal flow between valves. A short segment of reflux in the CFV opposite an incompetent SFj and in the popliteal vein opposite an incompetent SPj are not pathological deep reflux but simply the source feeding superficial reflux. We define deep reflux as being present if it extends beyond the valve below either junction. The amplitude and duration of deep reflux do not relate to the severity of varicose veins or risk of complications.

Venous occlusion can result from past venous thrombosis with incomplete or failed recanalization (Fig. 10.13). The degree to which flow is restricted depends on the extent of occlusion, where it is situated and the amount of collateral flow.

Other venous diseases

- **Haemangiomas** are localized superficial or deep congenital venous malformations that may be capillary, cavernous or diffuse.
- The **Klippel–Trenaunay syndrome** consists of varicose veins, haemangiomas, deep venous reflux and limb hypertrophy.
- **Left common iliac vein compression (May–Thurner syndrome)** occurs if the right common iliac artery compresses the left CIV as the artery becomes more rigid and tortuous with age (Fig. 10.14).

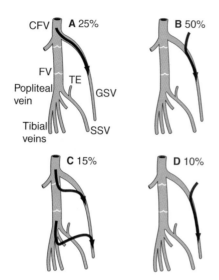

Fig. 10.12

Principal connections to the GSV system with residual or recurrent varicose veins from our studies

Sources for reflux are:

A: SFj or tributaries to the CFV
B: low pelvic or abdominal veins
C: perforators
D: unknown sources.

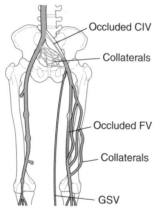

Fig. 10.13

Long standing occlusion of the FV or EIV and CIV

There is flow through collaterals or superficial veins.

Fig. 11.8 from Myers KA, Marshall RD and Freidin J. 1980: *Principles of Pathology*. Oxford: Blackwell. Reproduced with permission from Blackwell.

● **Popliteal vein entrapment** by the gastrocnemius muscle when the knee is extended can cause calf pain or predispose to deep vein thrombosis. However, it is also common in normal subjects.

● **Venous aneurysms** are uncommon but can affect the popliteal or femoral vein. They are saccular or fusiform and usually lined by thrombus, with a high risk of pulmonary embolism.

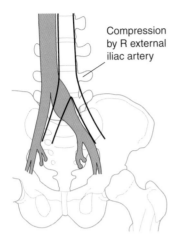

Compression
by R external
iliac artery

Fig. 10.14

Compression of the left CIV by the
right common iliac artery

Fig. 11.7a from Myers KA, Marshall RD
and Freidin J. 1980: *Principles of
Pathology*. Oxford: Blackwell.
Reproduced with permission from
Blackwell.

Clinical features

Patients present for cosmetic reasons or with symptoms that are not
necessarily proportional to the size of veins. Many symptoms are due
to conditions other than varicose veins. Athletes' prominent veins are
not a clinical problem. Large dilated veins can appear in pregnancy
and often regress after delivery.

Complications of chronic venous disease

Venous hypertension can damage skin and fat causing
lipodermatosclerosis that can lead to venous eczema or ulceration,
particularly at the ankle. Deep venous obstruction can cause 'venous
claudication' which is bursting pain in the calf during exercise
relieved by leg elevation. These complications are frequently referred
to as the 'post-thrombotic syndrome' implying that they are
inevitably a consequence of past DVT and recanalization or
obstruction, but duplex scanning has shown that many patients
develop complications from superficial reflux alone (see page 91 in
Chapter 5).

CEAP classification

This is used to characterize venous disease (Box 10.2).

Box 10.2: CEAP classification

C: **clinical** classification:
- C0: no visible or palpable signs of venous disease
- C1: telangiectases or reticular veins
- C2: varicose veins
- C3: oedema
- C4: skin changes ascribed to venous disease
  - a: pigmentation or eczema
  - b: lipodermatosclerosis or atrophy blanche
- C5: skin changes with healed ulcer
- C6: skin changes with active ulcer

E: **aetiological** classification:
- Ec: congenital problems apparent at birth or recognized later
- Ep: primary problems that are not congenital with no identifiable cause
- Es: secondary problems that are acquired with known pathology such as post-thrombotic or post-traumatic

A: **anatomical** classification:
- As: superficial veins
  - 1: telangiectases and reticular veins
  - 2: GSV above knee
  - 3: GSV below knee
  - 4: SSV
  - 5: non-saphenous
- Ad: deep veins
  - 6: IVC
  - 7: CIV
  - 8: IIV
  - 9: EIV
  - 10: pelvic – gonadal, broad ligament
  - 11: CFV
  - 12: PFV
  - 13: FV
  - 14: popliteal
  - 15: crural – ATV, PTV, peroneal
  - 16: Muscular – gastrocnemial, soleal, other
- Ap: perforator veins
  - 17: thigh
  - 18: calf

P: **pathophysiological** classification:
- Pr: reflux
- Po: obstruction
- Pro: both

Differential diagnosis

- Aching pain with walking or ulceration due to occlusive arterial disease.
- Swelling from lymphoedema.
- Skin changes from cellulitis.

Treatment

Treatment is directed towards destroying diseased surface veins.

- **Surgery** is effective, particularly for extensive collections of large veins.
- **Injection sclerotherapy** may be preferred for legs without saphenous reflux or residual and recurrent veins after surgery.
- **Ultrasound-guided sclerotherapy** can be used for large veins due to saphenous reflux (see page 313 in Chapter 16).
- **Endovenous techniques** can ablate the saphenous vein by a probe linked to a laser or radiofrequency heat source (see page 316 in Chapter 16).
- **Conservative treatment** with compression stockings may be the first or only option for complications.

The most common operation for either saphenous vein is to combine:

- **ligation** at the saphenous junction including all tributaries in the region
- **stripping** a length of saphenous vein
- **avulsion** of varicose veins through multiple tiny punctures.

Owing to proximity to surface sensory nerves, many limit stripping to the GSV between the groin and knee and the SSV just behind the knee.

What the doctors need to know

The examination should demonstrate patterns of anatomical abnormalities. Referrals come from surgeons, non-surgical phlebologists or general practitioners. They require the following information:

- are there sites of refluxing connections from deep to superficial veins through the saphenous junctions, incompetent perforators or other veins?
- is there superficial venous reflux in the GSV or SSV and their tributaries?
- what is the extent of GSV or SSV affected by reflux?
- is the SPj is present and what is its level?
- is there reflux in veins such as the TE, vein of Giacomini or gastrocnemius veins?
- is there deep venous reflux or obstruction?
- what are the diameters of incompetent saphenous junctions, saphenous veins and perforators?

Diameters have become important to help select the best treatment. Reflux in smaller diameter veins can be successfully treated by ultrasound-guided sclerotherapy whereas reflux in larger diameter veins may be better treated by surgery or other endovenous techniques.

Note!

Surface varicose veins affecting tributaries can be seen and it is not necessary to describe them in detail by duplex scanning.

THE DUPLEX SCAN

Normal findings

Reflux is flow in veins away from the heart and is normally prevented by valves. There is transient reflux for ≤0.5 s as a normal valve closes.

Alignment sign

The GSV and AASV can be distinguished by ultrasound from their relation to the femoral artery and vein (Fig. 10.15).

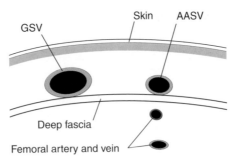

Fig. 10.15

Alignment sign in the left lower limb

The AASV lies superficial to the femoral artery and vein whereas the GSV is more medial.

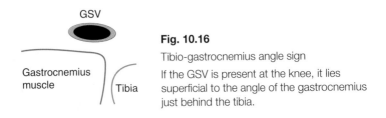

Fig. 10.16

Tibio-gastrocnemius angle sign

If the GSV is present at the knee, it lies superficial to the angle of the gastrocnemius just behind the tibia.

'Tibio-gastrocnemius angle sign'

Whether or not the GSV is present at the knee level can be determined by ultrasound (Fig. 10.16).

Indications for duplex scanning

If treatment is being considered:

● **primary uncomplicated great saphenous territory varicose veins:** scanning is recommended since clinical assessment alone will miss up to 30 per cent of important connections from deep to superficial veins when compared with duplex scanning

- primary uncomplicated small saphenous territory varicose veins: scanning is essential to determine whether there is a SPj, record its level, and show complex anatomy such as its relation to the TE, vein of Giacomini and gastrocnemius veins
- recurrent varicose veins: scanning is essential given that the anatomy is frequently complex
- chronic venous disease with skin complications: scanning is essential to detect the relative contributions of superficial and deep disease
- symptoms of venous disease without evidence of varicose veins: scanning is recommended since at least one-third show venous reflux
- surveillance after treatment: scanning is warranted given the frequency of recurrence
- venous malformations should be scanned to demonstrate the anatomy
- mapping the course of saphenous veins, level of the SPj and sites of perforators may be required prior to surgery for varicose veins
- mapping the course and diameters of saphenous veins may be required prior to their use for femoropopliteal or coronary artery bypass grafting.

Criteria for venous reflux

The original definition of reflux was reverse flow for $>0.5\,s$, but many consider that reflux for $>1\,s$ is required.

Note!

Testing for reflux is initiated by squeezing blood up through the deep system from the calf muscle plexus. Reflux is then detected into superficial veins. It follows that all varices should show deep to superficial connections but this is not possible in approximately 10 per cent.

PROTOCOLS FOR SCANNING

Follow the principles for venous scanning described on page 40 in Chapter 2.

Prepare the patient

Ask about past deep vein thrombosis, pregnancies and previous surgery. Ensure there is sufficient light in the room to be able to see the varicose veins. Examine the leg for the site of varicosities to help predict the source of reflux. Medial thigh and calf varices suggest SFj incompetence, posterior calf varices suggest SPj incompetence, and localized 'bunches' may be due to incompetent perforators. Look for scars from surgery as this may be the only way to determine whether the GSV or SSV have been previously ligated or excised. Check to see if there are skin changes from lipodermatosclerosis, eczema or ulceration and look to see where to avoid placing your hand for distal compression. Explain to the patient what is going to be done, particularly the Valsalva manoeuvre (see Box 10.3).

Note!

Reflux is more likely to develop later in the day and in a warm environment. A cold environment can cause veins to constrict and make them difficult to see, and in some cases causes refluxing veins to apparently become competent. These may change results of scans in patients with borderline reflux.

Select the best transducer

Both superficial and deep veins are best imaged with a medium- to high-frequency linear array transducer. Even higher frequency transducers may be used to show superficial varices. A lower frequency curved array transducer may be required to scan an obese or oedematous limb, deep veins in the thigh, particularly the FV at the adductor hiatus, or peroneal veins. Curved or phased array transducers are required if the examination involves iliac, pelvic or ovarian veins.

> **Warning!**
>
> Transducer pressure should remain light to ensure that superficial veins are not compressed making it difficult for them to be seen, or causing incompetent veins to become apparently competent. Do not be afraid to rest your scanning arm on the patient so that transducer pressure can be kept light without causing sonographer muscle strain.

Examination techniques to show reflux

Scan both limbs at the first examination. The leg being examined must be relaxed and dependent to allow good venous filling in calf muscle plexuses. The skin position in relation to veins changes with movement from upright to supine. If veins are being marked with an indelible pen prior to vein stripping or arterial bypass grafting, this should be performed with the patient supine and limb in the operation position.

Augmentation to test for reflux can be induced by:

- release after a thigh or calf squeeze for proximal veins, or calf or foot squeeze for calf veins
- manual compression of varicose vein clusters
- pneumatic calf cuff deflation
- active foot dorsiflexion and relaxation
- the Valsalva manoeuvre.

Box 10.3: The Valsalva manoeuvre*

This results from forced expiration against a closed glottis. The patient is asked to take a deep breath and then strain for a few seconds while holding the breath.

*Antonio Maria Valsalva (1666–1723), an Italian anatomist.

Veins above the knee
Position the patient

Scan with the patient standing, facing towards you with the leg rotated outwards, heel on the ground and weight taken on the opposite limb.

Use a frame for support if necessary. Alternatively, position the patient tilted on a table in reverse Trendelenburg to >45°.

Tips!

- The best way to assess varicose veins is to initially ignore varicosities and scan for sites of incompetence feeding to these veins. Only if this fails to show connections should varices be traced back to the saphenous veins.
- To minimize scan time, look for perforators while testing for deep and superficial reflux.
- Test for reflux in the CFV, femoral confluence and popliteal vein. It is not necessary to examine other deep veins if these are normal and there are no specific indications such as oedema, skin complications or previous DVT.

Scanning techniques for veins above the knee

GSV above the knee

- Commence in the groin in transverse to show the SFj and CFV as the 'Mickey Mouse image' (Fig. 2.1A, page 34). If the junction is not present due to ligation of the GSV then 'Mickey's' medial ear is missing.
- If present, determine the source of reflux by spectral or colour Doppler, from SFj incompetence, veins from the low abdomen or pelvis, thigh or calf perforators, or vein of Giacomini. We prefer to elicit reflux by the Valsalva manoeuvre (Fig. 10.17).
- In transverse, determine whether the destination for reflux is into the GSV or major thigh tributaries. Measure the level of inflow of reflux to the GSV if it is distal to the SFj.
- Scan for saphenous reflux distal to communication with a significant tributary (diameter > 4 mm).
- Suspect a source of reflux if there is a sudden increase in GSV diameter, whereas diameters decrease below major refluxing tributaries.
- Follow the full length of the GSV and tributaries to the knee. Test every few centimetres for compressibility and reflux.
- Measure diameters at the junction and along the GSV if there is reflux.

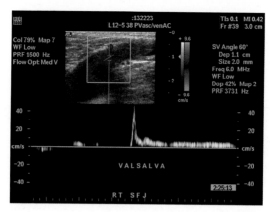

Fig. 10.17

Spectral Doppler for reflux at the SFj produced by the Valsalva manoeuvre

Deep veins in the thigh

● Test the CFV in longitudinal for phasicity with normal respiration, cessation of flow with deep inspiration and reflux with the Valsalva manoeuvre. Lack of phasicity may indicate proximal obstruction and the test should later be extended to show the iliac veins and IVC.

● If deep venous disease is suspected, follow the full length of FV to the above-knee popliteal vein testing for reflux and thrombus (see page 188 in Chapter 9). Move to an anterior window through the vastus medialis at the adductor hiatus if necessary.

● Slow outflow during distal compression suggests occlusion between the test and augmentation sites.

Thigh perforators

● Use colour Doppler to test for outward flow in perforators by thigh muscle contraction. Use spectral Doppler if flow direction and duration are ambiguous.

● Look for perforators on the medial thigh as the full length of the GSV and deep veins are examined.

● Look for lateral, posterior and anterior thigh perforators if clinical assessment shows varices in these regions.

● Measure the levels of refluxing perforators from the inguinal ligament or skin crease behind the knee.

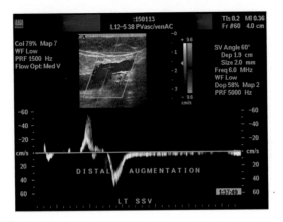

Fig. 10.18

Spectral Doppler for reflux at the SPj produced by augmentation

Antegrade flow in the SSV with calf compression followed by retrograde flow after release of calf compression.

Popliteal vein, SSV, TE and vein of Giacomini

Position the patient

Scan these veins with the patient standing and facing away with the knee slightly bent, heel on the ground and weight taken on the opposite limb, or prone in reverse Trendelenburg >45°.

Scanning techniques for SSV, TE and vein of Giacomini

- Start at the back of knee. Determine whether the SPj is present. If so, show the junction in longitudinal. Test the popliteal vein proximal and distal to the SPj, gastrocnemius veins insertion and SPj for reflux and thrombosis. Determine if there is SPj incompetence with SSV reflux (Fig. 10.18).
- Look for alternative sources of reflux including communication with popliteal fossa perforators, GSV tributaries, pelvic veins traced to the buttock or perineum, TE or vein of Giacomini.
- Look for alternative destinations for SSV reflux including tributaries, TE or vein of Giacomini.
- Examine the TE and vein of Giacomini. Determine the distal SSV connection and proximal connection into the GSV, deep or pelvic veins.

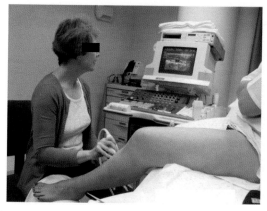

Fig. 10.19

Our preferred positioning of the patient to scan veins below the knee

- If there is reflux, measure diameters at the SPj and along the SSV, TE and vein of Giacomini.
- Measure the level of the SPj in relation to the skin crease behind the knee.
- Note whether the SSV is in the midline and measure its distance from the midline if it is medial or lateral.

Veins below the knee

Position the patient

Scan for below-knee veins with the patient standing facing towards you, sitting with the foot dependent on the examiner's knee (Fig. 10.19), or supine in reverse Trendelenburg >45°.

Scanning techniques for veins below the knee

Crural veins

- With experience, all crural veins can be identified. Reflux in the PTV best reflects clinical features. It is optional to scan the ATV.
- Examine the PTV from a medial or posteromedial view, the peroneal vein from a posteromedial or posterior view, and the ATV from an anterolateral view as described for crural arteries (Figs 8.25, page 171, and 8.26, page 172).

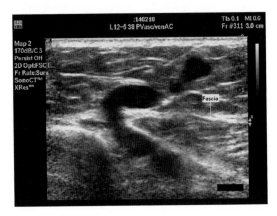

Fig. 10.20
A calf perforator passing through the deep fascia shown by B-mode

GSV below the knee

- Determine whether the below-knee GSV is present.
- Continue down its length as for the above-knee GSV.
- Examine for reflux and thrombosis.

Calf perforators

- Perforators pass through the deep fascia which is a distinct hyperechoic band on B-mode (Fig. 10.20).
- Test for outward flow by colour Doppler after a calf muscle squeeze, isometric calf muscle contraction or foot squeeze. Wait for >15 s to allow calf muscles to refill before repeating the squeeze. Use spectral Doppler if flow direction and duration is ambiguous with colour Doppler (Fig. 10.21).
- Look for perforators around the calf circumference. If they show outward flow, measure their diameters at the deep fascia, and level from the medial or lateral malleolus.

Note!

Insonate the fascia at 90° to ensure maximum specular reflection to help identify perforators passing through the fascia.

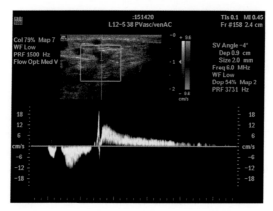

Fig. 10.21

Outward flow in a calf perforator shown by spectral Doppler.

Iliac and ovarian veins

Scanning these veins is usually left until last if performed at all. See Fig. 9.1 on page 182 for the anatomy of ovarian veins.

Position the patient and select the best window

The patient lies supine on a tilt table with >45° reverse Trendelenburg.

Scanning techniques for iliac and ovarian veins

- Iliac veins usually have no valves. Reflux may be detected into tributaries of the IIV or EIV. Ovarian vein reflux, usually on the left, may be the source for reflux through pelvic veins in many women.
- For the left side, find the left renal vein as it crosses superficial to the aorta and deep to the superior mesenteric artery, and trace it out to where it is joined by the left ovarian vein passing vertically upwards.
- For the right side, find the IVC and trace it down to where the right ovarian vein joins it at an anterior oblique and upwards direction.
- Test for reflux, either spontaneous or induced by epigastric compression. If spontaneous reflux is observed, this can be arrested by iliac fossa compression.

- If ovarian vein reflux is demonstrated, measure diameters in the proximal and distal segments.
- Use colour Doppler to scan the pelvic floor looking for varicosities.
- Test the IIV for incompetence.

Recurrent varicose veins

These are the most difficult studies for varicose veins. Patterns of reflux are frequently different from primary varicose veins so be aware of the many possible sites. If there has been previous surgery to the GSV, examine the medial and posterior thigh for recurrence of a refluxing GSV and source of reflux from the CFV, pelvic, round ligament, gluteal, abdominal, ovarian or pudendal tributaries, or thigh perforators. Examine the leg for recurrence through calf perforators. After past surgery to the SSV, examine the popliteal fossa for connections at the SPj, from popliteal or posterior calf perforators or from the TE or vein of Giacomini.

Surveillance after treatment for varicose veins

If the GSV and SSV are present, they should be examined throughout their lengths for thrombus, sclerosis or reflux. Scanning should include a complete DVT examination.

OTHER INVESTIGATIONS

The continuous-wave (CW) Doppler examination

The hand-held CW Doppler can be used to assess each GSV and SSV system and deep veins. Many doctors consider this to be a routine part of the clinical examination.

For the GSV:

- stand the patient facing you with the knee slightly bent, heel on the ground and weight taken on the opposite leg
- listen in the groin for the common femoral artery pulse. Move the probe a little medially to listen for reflux in the CFV after squeezing the calf
- move the probe a little more medial and down to be over the GSV and listen for reflux after squeezing the calf. If there is reflux,

then repeat and use a finger of the free hand to occlude the GSV below the probe to determine whether this stops reflux

- repeat listening over a distal varicosity to determine whether there is reflux and whether this can be stopped by pressure over the GSV. To detect whether a varicosity and the GSV are connected, push on one while listening over the other with the CW transducer to hear if there is a signal.

For the SSV:

- stand the patient on a step facing away with the knee slightly bent, heel on the step and weight on the opposite leg
- sit behind the patient and listen for the popliteal artery signal. Move the probe to the SSV just lateral to the arterial signal, squeeze the calf and listen for reflux after releasing the squeeze
- if there is reflux, repeat and use a finger of the free hand to occlude the SSV below the probe to determine whether this stops reflux.

Box 10.4: Ultrasound images to record

- Demonstrate incompetence or reflux by spectral Doppler for hard copy and colour Doppler for video.
- Sample spectral tracings of proximal veins and SFj in longitudinal with the Valsalva manoeuvre.
- Sample spectral tracings of more distal veins and SPj in longitudinal during augmentation and release.
- Reflux in other veins such as the TE, vein of Giacomini and gastrocnemius veins.
- B-mode for maximum and minimum vein diameters in transverse if reflux is demonstrated at either junction or in either saphenous vein.
- B-mode for diameters at the fascial border in transverse if there is outward flow in perforators.
- Other pathology such as a Baker's cyst.

11

DISEASES OF VESSELS TO THE UPPER LIMBS

Arterial disease is less common in the upper than in the lower limbs and the causes are more varied. Venous thrombosis occurs but venous reflux is rarely a clinical problem in upper limbs. Ultrasound is a good technique to screen for disease but most patients with arterial disease or venous thrombosis undergo angiography to help determine its site and extent. This approach is different from that for lower limb arterial disease where arteriography is usually performed only if intervention is contemplated.

ANATOMY

Box 11.1: Vessels scanned for reporting

- Subclavian artery and vein
- Axillary artery and vein
- Brachial artery and vein
- Radial artery and vein
- Ulnar artery and vein
- Basilic and cephalic veins

Other vessels discussed

- Superior vena cava: SVC
- Innominate artery and veins
- Palmar arches
- Antecubital vein

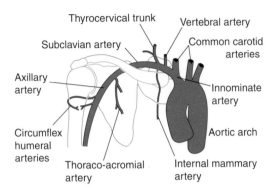

Fig. 11.1

Anterior view of arteries at the right thoracic outlet and axilla

- The innominate artery is the first branch of the aortic arch.
- The subclavian artery becomes the axillary artery as it leaves the thoracic outlet bounded by the first rib, scapula and clavicle.
- The internal mammary (thoracic) artery passes distally behind the cartilages of the first six ribs.

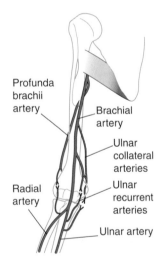

Fig. 11.2

Anterior view of arteries in the right arm

The axillary artery becomes the brachial artery passing to the elbow where it bifurcates.

Variations in vascular anatomy are more frequent in the upper than in the lower limb. The arterial supply is illustrated in Figs 11.1–11.3 and the venous drainage in Figs 11.4–11.5.

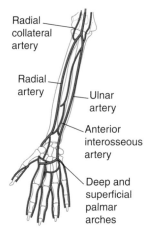

Radial collateral artery

Radial artery

Ulnar artery

Anterior interosseous artery

Deep and superficial palmar arches

Fig. 11.3

Anterior view of arteries in the right forearm

The radial artery is lateral and the ulnar artery is medial down to the hand where they join to form the palmar arches.

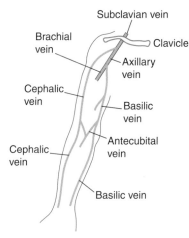

Subclavian vein

Brachial vein

Clavicle

Axillary vein

Cephalic vein

Basilic vein

Antecubital vein

Cephalic vein

Basilic vein

Fig. 11.4

Venous outflow in the right arm

Superficial venous outflow is through the basilic and cephalic veins, while deep venous drainage mirrors the arterial supply.

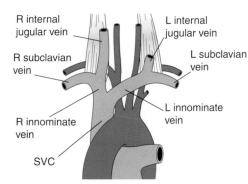

R internal jugular vein

L internal jugular vein

R subclavian vein

L subclavian vein

R innominate vein

L innominate vein

SVC

Fig. 11.5

Deep veins in the neck

The subclavian veins join the internal jugular veins to form the innominate veins which join to form the SVC.

CLINICAL ASPECTS

Regional pathology

Intrinsic arterial diseases

Atherosclerosis and degenerative aneurysms

Occlusive arterial disease can occur at any level. Proximal upper limb atherosclerosis frequently remains asymptomatic because of abundant collaterals around the shoulder. Severe innominate or subclavian artery disease can lead to reverse flow in the vertebral artery as a collateral to the arm for the 'subclavian steal syndrome' (see page 109 in Chapter 6). Innominate or subclavian artery aneurysms are not uncommon.

Autoimmune arteritis

Inflammatory arterial diseases are described on page 88 in Chapter 5. They can affect branches of the aortic arch to cause upper limb or cerebrovascular ischaemia, or they may affect more distal arteries to cause digital ischaemia. They include:

- Takayasu's disease
- Buerger's disease
- giant cell arteritis
- polyarteritis
- Behçet's syndrome
- scleroderma
- hypersensitivity reaction
- systemic lupus erythematosis.

Other intrinsic diseases

Fibromuscular dysplasia similar to that in the renal or carotid arteries, or cystic adventitial necrosis similar to that in the popliteal artery have been reported in the brachial artery.

Embolism

Some 10–20 per cent of emboli lodge in upper extremity arteries, most often in the brachial artery, less often the subclavian or axillary arteries and uncommonly in arteries below the elbow. The larger proportion comes from the heart but one-third originate from innominate or subclavian artery disease.

Repetitive external trauma

Thoracic outlet syndrome (TOS)

The subclavian artery, subclavian vein or brachial plexus can be compressed at the thoracic outlet. Arterial compression can cause turbulent flow, post-stenotic dilatation, intimal disruption, aneurysm formation, thrombosis and embolism (Fig. 11.6). The vein can be compressed leading to deep vein thrombosis: the **Paget–Schroetter syndrome**.

Bony or muscular abnormalities causing thoracic outlet compression

- The **cervical rib** or its fibrous extension runs along the anterior border of the scalenus medius muscle immediately under the artery. It is present in less than 1 per cent of individuals, 50 per cent are bilateral and fewer than 10 per cent cause symptoms.
- **Congenital abnormalities of the first rib** are less common than cervical rib, the most frequent being first rib atresia leaving an exostosis on the second rib at the scalenus anterior insertion.

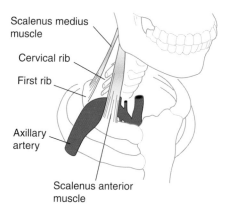

Fig. 11.6

Thoracic outlet syndrome

Subclavian artery compression can cause a post-stenotic axillary artery aneurysm.

Redrawn from Fig. 6.1 from Myers KA, in: Chant ADB and Barros D'Sa AAB (eds). 1997: *Emergency Vascular Practice*. London: Hodder Arnold.

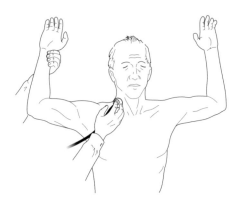

Fig. 11.7

'Military brace' manoeuvre

Opening and closing the hands 20 times causes pallor of the hand, loss of the radial pulse, and a bruit at the base of the neck if the artery is compromised.

Redrawn from Fig. 6.2 from Myers KA, in: Chant ADB and Barros D'Sa AAB (eds). 1997: *Emergency Vascular Practice*. London: Hodder Arnold.

- **Fibrosis of the scalenus anterior and medius muscles** can cause compression where the neurovascular bundle passes over the clavicle.
- **A previously fractured clavicle** can impinge on the artery.

Examination for vascular compression from the TOS is best performed by the 'military brace' manoeuvre (Fig. 11.7). It has a high incidence of false-positive results in normal subjects, but a negative test virtually excludes vascular involvement while a positive test provides confidence to proceed with treatment if there is an appropriate history.

External trauma around the shoulder

Throwing can cause injury to the axillary artery due to compression by the head of the humerus with the arm abducted and in external rotation. This has been studied in baseball pitchers, footballers, and field athletes.

External trauma to the hand and fingers

Repetitive catching or striking a ball with the hand can cause digital artery or palmar arch thrombosis. The '**hypothenar hammer** syndrome' can occur in workers who hammer with their hands. The ulnar artery is damaged just beyond the canal under the hamate bone causing acute thrombosis or aneurysm formation. Use of vibrating tools can cause distal small artery vasospasm or occlusion leading to the 'white finger syndrome'.

Iatrogenic trauma

Causes specific to the upper extremity include:

- brachial artery catheterization for arteriography or haemodynamic monitoring
- anaesthetic arm block with accidental intramural injection
- thrombosed axillofemoral bypass
- arteritis after radiotherapy for carcinoma of the breast
- harvesting the radial artery for coronary artery bypass grafting if it is the dominant artery to the hand.

Haematological disorders

Upper limb deep vein thrombosis is usually due to TOS. Thrombosis can result from a hypercoagulable state (see page 79 in Chapter 5) but this is far less common in upper than lower limbs, probably owing to lower venous pressures and less venous stasis. The risk of pulmonary embolism from upper limb deep vein thrombosis is less than from the lower limbs.

Raynaud's syndrome

Primary Raynaud's disease is vasospasm affecting the fingers due to abnormal sensitivity of vasomotor nerve endings. Arteriolar spasm is induced by cold or emotional disturbance, particularly in young females. **Secondary Raynaud's phenomenon** from scleroderma or other inflammatory artery diseases is more severe and persistent, and there is less sex or age difference.

Clinical presentations

- Mild to moderate ischaemia causing forearm fatigue or claudication.
- Raynaud's phenomenon with colour changes: pallor then cyanosis and rubor.

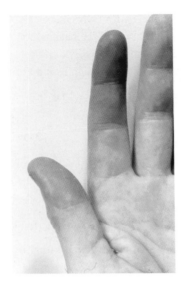

Fig. 11.8
Blue finger from ischaemia

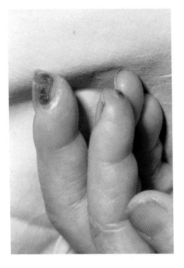

Fig. 11.9

Trophic changes in the finger tips due
to secondary Raynaud's disease

- Microemboli or occlusive disease causing the 'blue finger
  syndrome' (Fig. 11.8).
- Secondary Raynaud's disease causing trophic damage to the
  fingers or hands (Fig. 11.9).

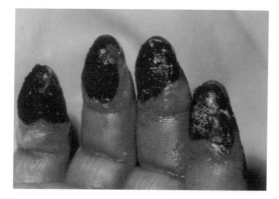

Fig. 11.10
Gangrene of the finger tips

- Severe ischaemia leading to gangrene (Fig. 11.10).
- Palpable aneurysm.
- Venous obstruction with oedema, cyanosis and visible collateral superficial veins.

Treatment

Occlusive or aneurysmal disease

Surgical bypass or endarterectomy may be required (Figs 11.11–11.13). Endovascular techniques using stenting or stent grafting are now widely used.

Thoracic outlet syndrome

Treatment usually involves removing the first rib and cervical rib, dividing all scalene muscle attachments and fibromuscular bands. Cervical sympathectomy may also be performed. An arterial aneurysm may require reconstruction. Venous thrombosis can be treated by thrombectomy or thrombolysis.

Embolism

Embolism is treated by embolectomy through the brachial artery at the elbow.

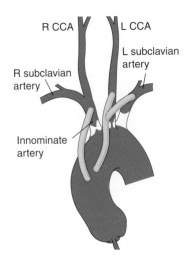

Fig. 11.11

Transthoracic synthetic bypass grafting from the aorta to major branches

Redrawn from Fig. 6.6 from Myers KA, in: Chant ADB and Barros D'Sa AAB (eds). 1997: *Emergency Vascular Practice*. London: Hodder Arnold.

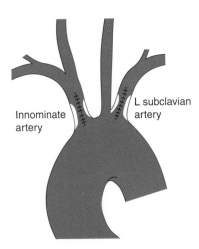

Fig. 11.12

Transthoracic innominate or left subclavian endarterectomy

Redrawn from Fig. 6.5 from Myers KA, in: Chant ADB and Barros D'Sa AAB (eds). 1997: *Emergency Vascular Practice*. London: Hodder Arnold.

What the doctors need to know

● Is there stenosis, occlusion, aneurysmal disease or vasospastic disease, and what is the nature of the pathology?

● Are there Doppler signal changes and a fall in arm pressures with the 'military brace' manoeuvre to reveal TOS?

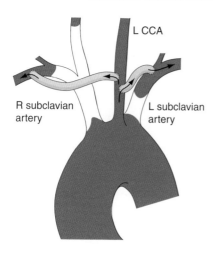

L CCA

R subclavian artery

L subclavian artery

Fig. 11.13

Extrathoracic common carotid to subclavian artery synthetic bypass

Redrawn from Fig. 6.8 from Myers KA, in: Chant ADB and Barros D'Sa AAB (eds). 1997: *Emergency Vascular Practice*. London: Hodder Arnold.

- Which is the dominant artery to the hand, prior to deciding whether to use the radial artery as a bypass graft?
- Where does mapping show superficial veins for use as arterial bypass grafts?
- Is there occlusive disease in the palmar arch, metacarpal arteries or digital arteries?

CLINICAL ASPECTS: OTHER CONDITIONS

Arteriovenous fistula or graft for haemodialysis

Techniques

The operations provide a large vein for repeated needle punctures to divert blood to a dialysis machine in patients with renal failure. The anastomosis for an arteriovenous (AV) fistula may be to veins at the wrist (Fig. 11.14) or cubital fossa (Fig. 11.15). Various methods can be used to join the artery and vein (Fig. 11.16). Alternatively, they can be connected by a vein or synthetic graft, usually PTFE (Fig. 11.17). It is best to form the AV fistula or graft in the non-dominant arm but it may be necessary to use the dominant arm or lower extremity (Fig. 8.19, page 160).

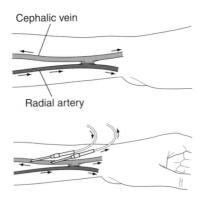

Fig. 11.14

Side-to-side AV fistula at the wrist

A: The preferred technique is to anastomose the cephalic vein to radial artery.

B: The vein is punctured to allow flow to the dialysis machine and back to the patient.

Fig. 7.11 from Uldall R. 1988: *Renal Nursing*. Oxford: Blackwell. Reproduced with permission.

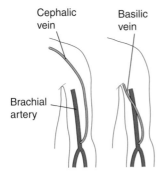

Fig. 11.15

End-to-side AV fistula at the cubital fossa

Anastomosis can be to the cephalic or basilic vein.

Figs 7.14 and 7.15 from Uldall R. 1988: *Renal Nursing*. Oxford: Blackwell. Reproduced with permission.

Fistula and graft maturation

There is a phase lasting approximately six weeks when the vein 'matures' to become large enough to allow repeated needling. The efferent vein may not mature if:

- there are vein tributaries
- a perforating vein steals flow from the superficial vein
- venous outflow is inadequate
- the vein is too deep to cannulate.

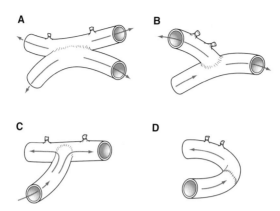

Fig. 11.16

Techniques for AV anastomosis

A: Side-to-side.
B: End of vein to side of artery.
C: End of artery to side of vein.
E: End-to-end.

Fig. 23.2 from Fahey V. 1994: *Vascular Nursing*. Philadelphia: WB Saunders. Reproduced with permission.

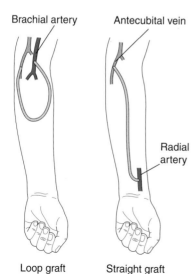

Fig. 11.17

Techniques for AV grafting for haemodialysis

Fig. 7.17 from Uldall R. 1988: *Renal Nursing*. Oxford: Blackwell. Reproduced with permission.

Complications

Complications include:

- thrombosis of the efferent vein or graft from repeated cannulations causing obstructed outflow
- anastomotic stenosis, usually due to neo-intimal hyperplasia but also from kinking hypoplasia or atherosclerotic plaque
- haematoma or false aneurysm
- perigraft fluid collection
- infection
- steal of arterial flow from the hand (Fig. 11.18).

Early detection of a failing graft allows correction before it occludes. Approximately one-third of asymptomatic patients have an abnormality which can be shown by ultrasound. Clinical features that suggest that the fistula or graft is failing or occluded are:

- failure of veins to dilate or mature
- elevation of venous pressures
- swelling of the arm
- poor flow for dialysis

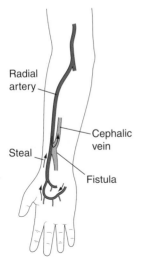

Radial artery

Steal

Cephalic vein

Fistula

Fig. 11.18

AV fistula steal

Flow may be away from the hand through the distal radial artery as well as flow into the vein from the proximal radial artery.

Redrawn from Fig. 6.12 from Myers KA, in: Chant ADB and Barros D'Sa AAB (eds). 1997: *Emergency Vascular Practice*. London: Hodder Arnold.

- reduction in the fistula 'thrill'
- palpable false aneurysm.

Treatment

Stenosis or thrombosis of a fistula or graft may require surgical revision, percutaneous balloon dilatation of percutaneous thrombolysis.

What the doctors need to know

- Are the arterial and venous systems suitable for construction of the fistula or graft?
- Can a fistula be formed or is a graft necessary?
- Where is the best site for the fistula or graft?
- Is the efferent vein maturing to allow haemodialysis?
- Is the fistula or graft remaining free from complications?

Mapping internal mammary vessels

The right and left internal mammary arteries (RIMA and LIMA) are frequently used as coronary artery bypass grafts. Ultrasound can be used to determine their presence and measure their length and diameter prior to operation and for surveillance of their continued patency after operation, when they adopt a characteristic coronary artery flow pattern with predominant flow in diastole.

In addition, internal mammary arteries and veins form the basis for maintaining viability for a free flap of skin, muscle and cartilage that can be used to replace a tissue defect for plastic surgery.

THE DUPLEX SCAN

The scan involves interrogating arteries from the aortic arch to wrist and veins through the upper extremity to the SVC. Scanning upper limb vessels can be challenging due to variations in anatomy and difficulties in negotiating the clavicle.

Normal findings

Upper limb arteries

Normal values for PSVs are not well established. Normal waveforms are triphasic but peripheral resistance decreases with arm exercise or warming the limb and hand causing the waveform to become monophasic with continuous flow through diastole. As skin temperature drops, waveforms remain triphasic but decrease in velocity.

Upper limb veins

- Deep inspiration increases venous flow (see page 75 in Chapter 4).
- The Valsalva manoeuvre decreases venous flow.
- There is full colour filling with distal augmentation.
- Pulsatile flow is seen in the internal jugular and innominate veins.
- There is phasic flow with respiration in proximal veins.
- Sudden sniffing causes momentary collapse of proximal veins and a brief increase in venous flow.
- Veins are compressible if they are accessible.

AV fistula or graft

To demonstrate that vessels are suitable for a dialysis fistula requires that:

- there are normal arteries with triphasic flow continuous from the major branches of the aortic arch to the wrist
- there is a continuous venous outflow pathway >3.5 mm diameter
- there is no venous thrombosis or wall thickening
- the vein is accessible for cannulation.

A fistula or graft has matured when the efferent vein has a diameter >3.5 mm over a length >3 cm.

Features of a normal functioning AV fistula or graft are:

- high PSV of 100–350 cm/s in the fistula or graft (Fig. 11.19)
- low-resistance spectral waveform with spectral broadening in the fistula or graft
- low-resistance waveform in the afferent artery and pulsatile flow in the efferent vein
- wall thickening of the vein adjacent to the fistula or graft anastomosis.

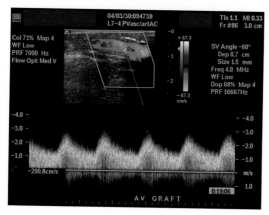

Fig. 11.19

A spectral tracing in a normal functioning AV graft for haemodialysis

Indications for scanning

● TOS with arterial, venous or neurological features.
● Major arterial disease causing forearm claudication or hand ischaemia.
● Raynaud's syndrome causing hand ischaemia.
● A pulsatile mass in the axilla.
● Arterial and venous mapping to select vessels suitable for a coronary artery bypass and lower limb arterial bypass grafts.
● Surveillance of a bypass graft.
● Assessment for suitability of arteries and veins for an AV fistula or graft.
● Assessment of the effect on the circulation to the hand prior to constructing an AV fistula or graft.
● Serial studies for maturation of an AV fistula or graft.
● Serial studies to detect complications in an AV fistula or graft.

Criteria for diagnosing disease

Upper limb arteries

Criteria for upper limb arterial stenosis are not well established. They are generally assumed to be the same as for lower limb arteries (see page 164 in Chapter 8). Criteria to define subclavian stenosis are discussed on page 110 in Chapter 6.

Upper limb veins

Thrombosis in major veins is diagnosed by:

- loss of compression if it can be elicited
- B-mode visualization of thrombus
- loss of flow with spectral or colour Doppler
- diminished flow, diminished or absent respiratory variations (Fig. 11.20), and diminished or absent response to the Valsalva manoeuvre or sniff test indicating proximal occlusion
- flow that does not increase with distal augmentation indicating obstruction between the transducer and augmentation site
- presence of collateral veins.

AV fistula or graft stenosis

Criteria used to diagnose stenosis or occlusion

Stenosis:

- PSV >400 cm/s or sudden increase in PSV ratio to 3:1 in the fistula or afferent artery
- PSV <50 cm/s in the efferent vein
- extreme turbulence in the efferent vein
- B-mode showing efferent vein diameter <3.5 mm (failure of maturation).

Stenosis or occlusion:

- decreased flow in the artery and vein
- pulsatile flow in the afferent artery but not in the efferent vein.

Occlusion:

- absence of flow with spectral and colour Doppler in the artery, vein or graft due to occlusion.

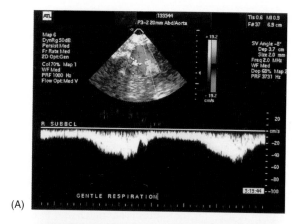

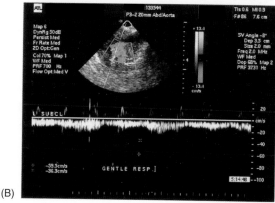

Fig. 11.20

Phasicity with respiration shown with spectral Doppler in a subclavian vein

A: Phasicity with respiration in the normal right subclavian vein.

B: Reduced phasicity with respiration distal to a partially thrombosed left subclavian vein.

A suspected failing fistula or graft should be evaluated by arteriography.

PROTOCOLS FOR SCANNING

Follow the techniques for scanning peripheral arteries and veins discussed on pages 38 and 40 in Chapter 2.

Prepare the patient

Ensure adequate access to the neck and arms. Ask when symptoms occur and their nature. Explain the provocative positions to assess TOS and find out what position brings on symptoms. Feel for pulses.

Select the best transducer

Use a medium-frequency linear array transducer to image vessels to the elbow. A high-frequency transducer may be required for good images of vessels distal to the elbow, the superficial basilic and cephalic veins, or for a slim arm. A phased array transducer with its small footprint is used for the suprasternal notch and to image deep vessels at the base of the neck.

Vessels in the thoracic outlet

Position the patient and select a window

For proximal vessels, examine the patient seated or standing so that the shoulder girdle is relaxed and falls down under gravity to improve access. Examine subclavian and axillary vessels through suprasternal, supraclavicular and infraclavicular windows. Use copious gel to maintain good skin contact in the suprasternal notch. The axillary artery is easier to see with the arm abducted and scanned from an axillary approach but it can be scanned through an anterior window. Examine both arms even if there are only unilateral symptoms.

Scanning techniques for vessels at the thoracic outlet

Provocative positions for TOS are:

- abduction to 90° or 180°
- 'military brace' position: arms elevated to 90° with the shoulders forced as far back as possible
- Adson's manoeuvre: arms dependent with the neck braced backwards and head turned to the ipsilateral side with the patient holding in a deep breath
- any position that brings on symptoms.

> ## Note!
>
> If there is excessive movement of vessels with respiration, ask the patient to hold the breath.

First, examine the **arteries**:

- with the arm dependent, use B-mode to measure the lumen diameter of the subclavian artery at the clavicle and note proximal arterial pathology if present
- use colour and spectral Doppler to demonstrate aliasing and obtain a sample trace in the proximal subclavian artery
- with the arm dependent, use colour Doppler to demonstrate aliasing and use spectral Doppler to measure PSV in the subclavian and axillary arteries at the clavicle. Note if post-stenotic turbulence is present
- repeat with the arm in different positions
- if a tight stenosis or occlusion is present in the subclavian artery, examine the ipsilateral vertebral artery for reverse flow
- note dampened and monophasic waveforms in the axillary artery distal to stenosis or external compression
- use B-mode to assess adjacent soft tissue and bony structures around the shoulder.

Then examine the **veins**:

- image the internal jugular vein from the base of neck to as high as possible in transverse, using B-mode to test for compressibility and spectral and colour Doppler for spontaneous colour filling, pulsatile flow and respiratory fluctuations
- have the patient perform the sniff test to see if the veins collapse, indicating that they are thrombus-free
- with the arm dependent, examine the subclavian and axillary veins in longitudinal and transverse to measure vein diameters, and assess flow patterns, compressibility and other pathology

- look for extrinsic venous compression with the arm in different positions
- examine the axillary vein to see if it is dilated due to proximal obstruction or occlusion.

Pitfalls!

- There can be a rich venous collateral system in the neck.
- Interference by bony structures can obscure proximal subclavian thrombus.
- Colour can obscure non-occlusive thrombus if colour gain and priority are set too high.
- A 90° insonation angle prevents colour-filling of vessels.
- Subclavian vessels can have a mirror image deep to the high-impedance mismatch of the pleura–lung interface.

Upper limb vessels beyond the thoracic outlet

Position the patient and select a window

With the patient upright, externally rotate the arm to view the brachial vessels from a medial window between the triceps and biceps muscles. For most distal arteries, it is easier to scan with the patient supine. For veins, examine the patient seated or standing to fill the veins for better identification. Use a venous tourniquet around the upper arm to dilate veins for pre- and post-operative assessment of an AV fistula or graft.

Scanning techniques for upper limb arteries

- Follow with colour Doppler and use spectral Doppler to record PSVs in major arteries in the arm and forearm, and note segments of stenosis or occlusion measured from the elbow or wrist.
- PSVs progressively fall the more distally you scan so continually decrease the colour scale to ensure adequate colour filling.

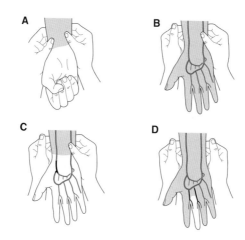

Fig. 11.21

Allen's test

A: The radial and ulnar arteries are compressed and the hand is exercised to produce ischaemia.

B: Normal – compression of one or both arteries is released and there is prompt reperfusion of the hand.

C: Radial artery occlusion – radial artery compression is released but there is no immediate reperfusion.

D: Metacarpal artery occlusions – arterial compression is released and all fingers reperfuse except the finger affected by disease.

Redrawn from Fig. 6.3 from Myers KA, in: Chant ADB and Barros D'Sa AAB (eds). 1997: *Emergency Vascular Practice*. London: Hodder Arnold.

- The radial artery is a more direct extension of the brachial artery than the ulnar artery.
- Record PSVs in the palmar arch and metacarpal arteries before and after compression of the radial and ulnar arteries as for Allen's test (Fig. 11.21).

Scanning techniques for upper limb veins

- Incompetence studies are not performed as upper limb varicose veins are rare.
- Scan the axillary, brachial, radial and ulnar, and cephalic and basilic veins for thrombosis (see page 188 in Chapter 9).

> ## Pitfalls!
>
> - A normal nerve is easily mistaken for a thrombosed brachial vein.
> - There may be duplicated brachial veins – ensure that both are identified.
> - Deep veins of the forearm are small and difficult to see.

Scanning techniques to assess suitability for an AV fistula or graft

- Use spectral Doppler to test for phasicity and pulsatility in the innominate, internal jugular and subclavian veins.
- Use colour Doppler with distal augmentation and compression testing in B-mode to determine the patency of all deep and superficial upper limb veins.
- Note the level of any tributaries and perforating veins that communicate with the cephalic or basilic veins and measure their level from the elbow crease. Ensure that the cephalic and basilic veins are superficial at all levels.
- In B-mode, measure diameters of the cephalic and basilic veins noting the location and extent from the elbow crease of any segment <3.5 mm diameter.
- Use colour and spectral Doppler to ensure patency of all upper limb arteries and to classify the degree of stenosis. Use B-mode to classify plaque type.

Scanning techniques for examining an AV fistula or graft

- Study on a day when there are no dressings applied.
- Examine with the patient lying and the arm by the side.
- Set the colour scale high to minimize colour Doppler aliasing in the high-flow circulation.
- Use B-mode to measure the lumen and graft diameters.
- Use colour Doppler to determine flow direction and detect stenosis.
- Commence with spectral Doppler in the distal brachial artery. Continue by 'walking' the spectral sample volume through the

afferent artery to the anastomosis, looking for stenosis or occlusion.

- Take a sample trace from the artery distal to the anastomosis to determine flow direction and detect steal.
- Adjust the cursor angle as the sample volume passes through the connection to the efferent vein and continue scanning to the subclavian vein.
- Measure diameters and assess patency of the cephalic or basilic, brachial, axillary and subclavian veins.
- Measure the length and note the location relative to the elbow crease of any segment of the efferent vein <3.5 mm diameter.
- Measure location of diameter reductions, thrombus, aneurysmal dilatation, and arterial stenosis or occlusion from the elbow crease.

Pitfalls!

- Shadowing may obscure full insonation of an AV graft
- The efferent vein of an AV fistula or graft is very superficial and care must be taken to prevent compression that might appear to show stenosis of the vein.
- The fistula or graft may have been placed in widely variable positions.

Scanning for the internal mammary arteries and veins

The patency, length, diameter and branching of these arteries and veins on each side need to be documented.

Scanning for arterial and venous mapping

- Use colour and spectral Doppler to determine patency and exclude stenosis in the radial arteries. Use B-mode to measure diameter and detect plaque.
- Use B-mode to determine patency, diameter, communication with perforators and tributaries of the superficial veins. Use B-mode for compression testing and colour Doppler with distal augmentation to detect thrombus or wall thickening in veins.

OTHER INVESTIGATIONS

Allen's test

This is used as a clinical test observing colour changes to determine the distribution of occlusive arterial disease in the hands and fingers (Fig. 11.21).

Continuous-wave Doppler, photoplethysmography or duplex ultrasound can be used to supplement clinical observation. The presence of flow and its direction are observed in the radial and ulnar arteries in the hand distal to active compression of each artery in turn at the wrist. The aims are to:

- detect occlusive arterial disease in the radial or ulnar artery, or the palmar arches and their branches, particularly with Raynaud's syndrome,
- determine whether the radial or ulnar artery is the dominant artery to the hand, prior to deciding whether to use the radial artery as a bypass graft to ensure that its removal does not cause hand ischaemia.

Pressure measurements

Use CW Doppler to measure pressures in the brachial, radial and ulnar arteries. A pressure difference >20 mmHg between sides at the same level indicates occlusive disease in the side with the lowest pressure. A pressure difference >20–30 mmHg between different levels of the same arm indicates occlusive disease in that segment. As with the lower limbs, heavily calcified arteries can cause spurious high pressure readings. Use CW Doppler to map out palmar arch, metacarpal and digital arteries.

> ## Warning!
>
> Do not inflate a cuff over an AV fistula or graft for fear of causing occlusion.

Photoplethysmography

- Ultrasound for TOS is complemented by recording digital arterial flow using photoplethysmography (PPG). Place a PPG sensor on the tip of the middle or index finger.
- Look for a diminished or absent trace with the arm in various positions for TOS.
- Look for a diminished or absent trace while performing Allen's test.

Box 11.2: Ultrasound images to record

- Sample traces from vessels listed in Box 11.1.

For arteries:

- spectral traces proximal to and at arterial stenoses
- B-mode for diameters of aneurysmal arterial dilatation and proximal and distal diameters of adjacent normal artery.

For veins:

- dual image representing a non-compressed and compressed vein (if bones are not hindering compression)
- spectral trace showing venous flow with normal spontaneous respiration and response to Valsalva manoeuvre or distal compression
- thrombus in veins detected in transverse and longitudinal with B-mode and colour Doppler noting whether it is occlusive or non-occlusive, whether recanalization is present, and its location and extent.

For TOS with arm dependent and in provocative positions:

- spectral traces and B-mode for diameters from the subclavian artery at the clavicle and axillary artery
- spectral traces and B-mode for diameters from subclavian and axillary veins with normal respiration and response to Valsalva manoeuvre or distal compression.

For preoperative assessment of an AV fistula or graft:

- sample spectral traces for all upper limb arteries
- sample spectral traces for proximal veins showing flow with normal respiration and response to Valsalva manoeuvre or distal compression
- dual B-mode images showing non-compressed and compressed upper limb and internal jugular veins (if bones are not hindering compression)
- B-mode diameters of cephalic and basilic veins noting the distance from a landmark if diameter is <3.5 mm.

For post-operative assessment of an AV fistula or graft:

- B-mode diameters of afferent artery, proximal mid and distal fistula or graft, and efferent vein
- sample spectral traces from these sites and the artery distal to the anastomosis
- spectral traces from any stenosis noting the location and extent.

12

RENOVASCULAR DISEASES

Ultrasound is used to screen for renovascular disease, or to help plan and follow the outcome of interventional treatment. Duplex scanning has no more than 95 per cent sensitivity and 90 per cent specificity for detecting renal artery stenosis when compared with digital subtraction angiography (DSA). However, contrast for DSA is nephrotoxic and carries a high risk of worsening renal function if it is already compromised. Other investigations such as computed tomographic angiography (CTA) or magnetic resonance angiography (MRA) may be preferred if the duplex scan is technically inadequate.

ANATOMY

Box 12.1: Vessels scanned for reporting

- Aorta
- Renal arteries and veins
- Segmental, interlobar, interlobular and arcuate arteries

Other vessels discussed

- Superior mesenteric artery: SMA
- Common iliac artery: CIA
- Internal iliac artery: IIA
- External iliac artery: EIA
- Inferior vena cava: IVC

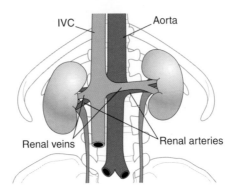

Fig. 12.1

Renal arteries

- Are paired at approximately the same level at the first to second lumbar vertebrae, just distal to the SMA.
- Arise at approximately right angles to the aorta, the left being more posterior than the right.
- Are frequently multiple, with accessory renal arteries from the aorta to the upper or lower poles of the kidney in 15 per cent.
- The right renal artery is longer than the left, and passes posterior to the IVC.
- The left renal artery has a more horizontal course to the kidney.

Renal veins

- Lie anterior to the renal arteries.
- The left renal vein is longer than the right and passes to the IVC between the aorta and SMA.
- Tributaries are the left gonadal, adrenal and posterior lumbar veins.

Renal arteries pass from the aorta to the renal hilum in the retroperitoneal plane just distal to the SMA, while renal veins pass to the IVC (Fig. 12.1). Arteries branch extensively at the hilum and within the kidney (Fig. 12.2).

CLINICAL ASPECTS

Regional pathology and clinical presentations

Renal artery stenosis or occlusion

Renal artery stenosis is usually caused by atherosclerosis (Fig. 12.3). Less frequently, stenosis is caused by fibromuscular

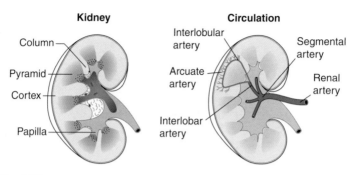

Fig. 12.2

Branches of each renal artery

- The renal artery divides into anterior and posterior branches near the hilum.
- There are five extrarenal segmental arteries: apical, upper, middle, lower and posterior.
- Each becomes a lobar artery that branches into interlobar and interlobular arteries between the renal pyramids.
- These terminate as arcuate arteries that course between the cortex and medulla.
- These terminate as glomerular arterioles.

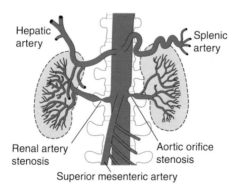

Fig. 12.3

Renal artery stenoses from atherosclerosis

Right: plaque in the proximal renal artery.

Left: plaque in the adjacent aorta (osteal stenosis).

Fig. 12.1d from Myers KA, Marshall RD and Freidin J. 1980: *Principles of Pathology*. Oxford: Blackwell. Reproduced with permission from Blackwell.

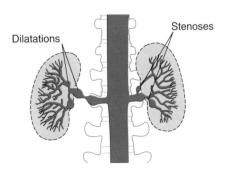

Fig. 12.4

Renal artery stenoses from fibromuscular dysplasia

Multiple stenoses and dilatations in mid to distal extrarenal arteries.

Fig. 12.1 and from Myers KA, Marshall RD and Freidin J. 1980: *Principles of Pathology*. Oxford: Blackwell. Reproduced with permission from Blackwell.

dysplasia (Fig. 12.4), particularly in women. Occlusion is usually due to thrombosis complicating atherosclerosis and rarely secondary to fibromuscular dysplasia. Collateral circulation to major branches can develop from non-renal sources. Renal artery disease is frequently asymptomatic but it can lead to secondary renal hypertension or progressive renal failure.

Renovascular hypertension

Decreased renal perfusion from renal artery disease can cause release of renin from endocrine cells in glomeruli. Renin is part of a feedback loop that regulates arterial blood pressure. Renin converts angiotensinogens to angiotensins and these directly increase systemic peripheral resistance. In addition, one angiotensin acts at the adrenal gland to stimulate aldosterone secretion to cause sodium and fluid retention. Both effects can lead to hypertension.

Nephropathy from intrarenal disease

Damage can result from ischaemia due to renal artery disease, or other primary renal diseases such as diabetic nephropathy, glomerulonephritis, pyelonephritis, acute tubular necrosis, analgesic nephropathy or hypertensive nephrosclerosis. These cause morphological and functional changes with diffuse or focal areas of reduced or absent perfusion leading to increased vascular resistance. Patients present with hypertension or have an elevated blood creatinine level. Renal failure develops when the amount of functioning renal tissue is reduced by approximately 80 per cent.

Renal vein thrombosis

Thrombosis of one or both renal veins or adjacent IVC can be spontaneous, secondary to haematological disturbance, or from extension of renal carcinoma. A retroperitoneal tumour or lymphadenopathy can cause extrinsic compression. The left renal vein can be compressed between the aorta and SMA – the '**nutcracker syndrome**'.

Presentation may be acute with a mass in the flank, haematuria or thrombocytopenia, or chronic as in the '**nephrotic syndrome**' with gross proteinuria and impaired renal function.

Treatment

Renovascular hypertension is initially managed by drug treatment. Intervention is required if hypertension remains uncontrolled or if there is progressive deterioration of renal function. This may lead to surgical endarterectomy or bypass grafting, but intervention for renal artery stenosis is now usually by balloon dilatation and stenting.

Progressive renal failure is initially treated by peritoneal dialysis or haemodialysis (see page 237 in Chapter 11). Kidney transplantation may be required for irreversible renal failure (Fig. 12.5).

What the doctors need to know

- Is there disease in renal arteries or veins and what is its location and severity?
- Is there disease in the kidneys or intrarenal circulation and what is its location and severity?
- Are there ultrasound changes over time with surveillance for untreated disease?

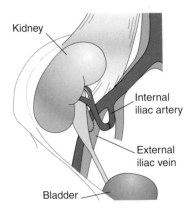

Fig. 12.5

Kidney transplantation

- Kidney placed in the iliac fossa.
- Anastomosis of renal artery end-to-end to the internal iliac artery or end-to-side to the common or external iliac artery or aorta.
- Anastomosis of renal vein to an iliac vein.

Redrawn from Fig. P457 of Scott R. 1982: *Urology Illustrated*. ©1982, with permission from Elsevier.

- Are there ultrasound changes with surveillance after renal artery balloon dilatation and stenting or renal transplantation?

THE DUPLEX SCAN

Box 12.2: Abbreviations

- PSV: peak systolic velocity (cm/s)
- RAR: renal–aortic ratio = $PSV_{renal\ artery}/PSV_{aorta}$
- EDV: end diastolic velocity (cm/s)
- EDR: end diastolic ratio = EDV/PSV.
- RI: resistance index = $(1 - EDV/PSV) \times 100$
- AT: acceleration time = time from onset to the early systolic peak (ms)
- AI: acceleration index = systolic upslope/transducer frequency $(cm/s^2)(KHz/s.MHz)$

Normal findings

> ### Box 12.3: Normal measurements from renal Duplex findings
>
> Arteries outside the kidney:
> - PSV: 50–150 cm/s
> - RAR: 0.5–1.5
> - EDV: <50 cm/s
>
> Arteries at the hilum:
> - AT: <100 ms
> - AI: >3.8 cm/s^2
>
> Intrarenal vessels:
> - EDR: >0.30
> - RI: <70
>
> B-mode – the kidney:
> - pole-to-pole length: >9 cm
> - width 4.5–6 cm
> - cortical thickness: 1–2 cm

Normal waveforms

Renal arteries supply low-resistance end organs so there is a blunted peak at systole and constant forward diastolic flow. Spectral broadening is noted if a wide sample volume is used. The PSV decreases as the renal arteries and branches are followed out to the kidneys. **Renal veins** have flow towards the IVC with some respiratory and cardiac fluctuations.

Indications for scanning

- Uncontrolled hypertension.
- Hypertension in young patients.
- Hypertension of rapid onset.
- Epigastric or flank bruit.
- Renal intervention surveillance.
- Kidney transplantation.

Assessment before intervention

Prior to balloon dilatation and stenting, it is important to know:

- whether disease is at the ostium or into the renal artery
- the angle of the renal artery to aorta
- whether there are accessory renal arteries.

These may require other imaging techniques.

Before kidney transplantation, the aorta, IVC and iliac arteries and veins should be scanned to ensure that they are of adequate diameter and not diseased.

Surveillance after treatment

Renal artery balloon dilatation and stenting requires post-operative surveillance since there is a poor correlation between restenosis and blood pressure control or deterioration of renal function. It is usual to scan post-procedure at one and six months and then annually.

Kidney transplant abnormalities that can be studied by ultrasound include:

- vascular abnormalities from renal artery or vein stenosis, thrombosis or compression, or false aneurysm
- functional abnormalities: ischaemic nephropathy causing acute tubular necrosis, acute and chronic rejection, and cyclosporin-induced nephropathy
- morphological abnormalities such as hydronephrosis and perirenal collections.

Criteria for diagnosing disease

Renal artery stenosis

Even expert sonographers detect only 80–90 per cent of renal arteries. Ultrasound contrast agents improve the technical success rate to >95 per cent. Power Doppler provides greater sensitivity for intrarenal vessels but is subject to flash artefact. Harmonic imaging, if available, aids B-mode identification of the renal arteries and kidneys.

Accessory renal arteries are rarely detected by ultrasound and are better shown by CTA or MRA. There is no consensus as to the best criteria for detecting critical renal artery stenosis or parenchymal disease. False-negative results may occur with fibromuscular dysplasia, branch artery stenoses, multiple renal arteries or impaired renal function.

Box 12.4: Criteria for renal artery stenosis (Fig. 12.6)

<60 per cent stenosis
Arteries outside the kidney:

- PSV >180cm/s
- no post-stenotic turbulence
- RAR 1.5–3.5.

>60 per cent stenosis
Arteries outside the kidney:

- PSV >180 cm/s
- post-stenotic turbulence
- RAR >3.5
- a distal dampened 'tardus parvus' spectral waveform.

Arteries at the hilum:

- AT >100 ms
- AI >3.7 cm/s^2

Colour Doppler demonstrates post-stenotic turbulence. PSVs may return to normal distal to a renal artery stenosis but often remain dampened. The RAR is preferred to PSV criteria unless the aortic PSV is <40 cm/s or >100 cm/s, or if there is an abdominal aortic aneurysm. The AT and AI (Fig. 12.6) were introduced as they are easier to measure than arterial PSVs since they are not angle-specific, but they have lower sensitivity for detecting renal artery disease and they cannot distinguish severe stenosis from occlusion.

Renal artery occlusion

- A clear view of the renal artery with no flow detected.
- Reduced parenchymal renal blood flow velocity <10 cm/s.

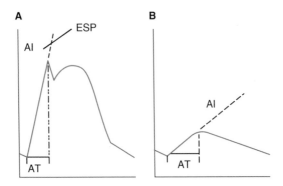

Fig. 12.6

Calculation of the renal artery acceleration time (AT) to the early systolic peak (ESP) and acceleration index (AI)

A: Normal signal.

B: The tardus-parvus renal artery signal (tardus: slowed systolic acceleration; parvus: low-amplitude systolic peak) with renal artery stenosis.

Reprinted from Fig. 2, Lavoipierre AM, Dowling AJ, Little AF. Ultrasound of the renal vasculature. *Ultrasound Quarterly* ©2000;**16**:123–132, with permission from Lipincott Williams and Wilkins, Philadelphia.

- A delayed AT at the hilum.
- A small kidney.
- Collateral flow.

Intrarenal arterial and parenchymal disease

Box 12.5: Criteria for intrarenal arterial and parenchymal disease

B-mode appearance of kidney:

- pole-to-pole length <8 cm and smaller than the contralateral kidney
- cortical hyperechogenicity on the B-scan.

Extrarenal Doppler characteristics:

- AT >100 ms

Intrarenal Doppler characteristics:

- EDR reduction:
- 0.25–0.30: minor
- 0.20–0.25: moderate
- <0.20: severe
- RI >80
- RI >5 per cent difference for a unilateral stenosis compared with the other side.

The AT may be normal with proximal renal artery stenosis if there is high resistance due to associated intrarenal disease. The EDR can assess the severity of intrarenal disease. Both PSV and the indices can be used for surveillance to measure the rate of disease progression. The pre-operative RI predicts improvement of blood pressure and renal function after renal artery balloon dilatation or stenting – RI > 80 indicates that treatment may be ineffective and RI < 80 predicts a good response.

Renal vein thrombosis

This is diagnosed if the renal vein is seen but no Doppler signal is detected. Other findings may be an intraluminal filling defect with colour Doppler, lack of venous flow in the parenchyma, an enlarged kidney, and dilated intrarenal veins and venous collaterals. The renal vein diameter is increased distal to compression with the 'nutcracker syndrome'.

Kidney transplantation

Ultrasound can screen for problems that are not yet clinically obvious or detect reasons for deteriorating renal function.

- A renal artery/common iliac artery PSV ratio >3.0 with post-stenotic turbulence is diagnostic for >60 per cent renal artery stenosis.
- Decreased diastolic flow and increasing RI and EDR with serial studies may indicate acute tubular necrosis, transplant rejection or cyclosporin toxicity before clinical features are apparent. A falling

RI is a good sign that acute tubular necrosis or rejection is recovering.

PROTOCOLS FOR SCANNING

Follow the techniques for abdominal scanning discussed on page 43 in Chapter 2.

Prepare the patient

The examination is most often successful in thin patients and children. Vessels may be obscured by obesity, intestinal gas, respiratory motion, abdominal aortic aneurysm, arterial calcification, or scarring from prior surgery. A scar in the right or left iliac fossa indicates the site of a transplant and a flank scar may indicate nephrectomy. The patient must be prepared with nil orally until one hour before the scan after which several glasses of water are taken (see page 51 in Chapter 3).

Select the best transducer

Commence with a low-frequency curved array transducer. Use the lower frequency small-footprint phased array transducer to allow angulation in several directions, including insonation between the ribs and bowel gas or for large patients.

Position the patient and select a window

It is technically difficult to scan renal vessels. Lay the patient supine with the head elevated on an examination table tilted 10–20° in reverse Trendelenburg to allow the viscera to descend slightly into the abdomen. Vary positioning if there is aortic aneurysmal dilatation or tortuosity or bowel gas.

- **Aorta and proximal renal arteries:** use an anterior window through the rectus abdominus muscles.
- **Mid to distal renal arteries and kidneys:**
  - for a slim, non-gassy patient, use the anterior approach, angling to right and left lateral views

- for a large or gassy patient, use a flank or intercostal approach with the patient in lateral decubitus.
- **Kidneys:** use a posterior or lateral window through the subcostal or intercostal spaces with the patient in lateral decubitus. Open the spaces by asking the patient to stretch the arm above the head and straighten the leg.

Scanning techniques for the aorta

- Commence imaging at the xiphoid process in longitudinal to evaluate the full length of the abdominal aorta. Note tortuosity, aneurysmal dilatation or arterial wall irregularity. Perform a full scan for an abdominal aortic aneurysm if detected (see page 167 in Chapter 8)
- Record spectral signals throughout the aorta. Record PSV in the suprarenal aorta at the level of the SMA in longitudinal to calculate the RAR.
- Image the aorta in transverse and work down to the left renal vein as it crosses anterior to the aorta and posterior to the SMA which is a reliable landmark to locate the renal arteries. The right renal artery is located at approximately 10 o'clock and the left renal artery at approximately 4 o'clock.

Scanning techniques for renal arteries and veins

- Increase the sweep speed to better define the systolic upstroke.
- Use colour Doppler to identify each renal artery as it arises from the lateral wall of the aorta just distal to the left renal vein.
- Begin in the aorta or renal hilum, keep the sample volume small, ask the patient to stop breathing for short intervals and 'walk' the spectral Doppler sample volume through the length of each renal artery and at its orifice.
- Record velocities at the origin, mid and distal segments or wherever a stenosis is detected.
- Look for multiple renal arteries.
- Look for renal vein thrombosis with no colour or spectral signal in the vein.

- Look for the 'nutcracker syndrome' with compression between the SMA and aorta and distal renal vein dilatation.

> **Tip!**
>
> The renal artery at the hilum is best identified by scanning the kidney in transverse.

Scanning techniques for the kidneys and intrarenal circulation

- Measure the pole-to-pole kidney length (Fig. 12.7). Look for increased cortical echogenicity.
- Use colour or power Doppler to identify the arteries and their branches (Fig.1.21, page 24). Make the sample volume large and turn off the angle facility as the only concern now is with Doppler waveform morphology and not velocities.
- Ask the patient to hold the breath to obtain waveforms from hilar segmental arteries, interlobar arteries, and upper and lower cortical interlobular arteries.

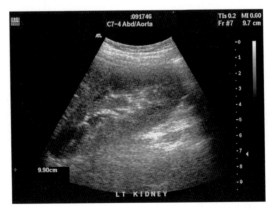

Fig. 12.7
B-mode image of kidney in longitudinal

- Use the advanced measurements facility to calculate AT and AI at the hilum. Calculate the EDR and RI for intrarenal arteries.
- Note non-vascular abnormalities such as cysts, tumours, hydronephrosis or calculi.

Scanning techniques for kidney transplants

- Examine the full lengh of the iliac arteries.
- Trace the renal artery from the anastomosis and then continue to examine as for a native renal artery study. Determine patency and measure PSV in the main renal artery and at the anastomosis. Determine patency of the vein. Note that end-to-side anastomosis can cause turbulence without increased velocities.
- The spectral waveform is normally high-resistance in the iliac arteries and their branches and low-resistance in the renal artery. If the anastomosis is to an external iliac artery, use this to distinguish the transposed renal artery from an iliac branch. If the anastomosis is to the internal iliac artery then it will also have a low-resistance signal.
- Examine the whole kidney to detect a focal or global decrease in parenchymal vascularity and calculate the RI from the upper, mid and lower portions of the transplant. Use B-mode to show kidney length and hydronephrosis or perirenal fluid collections and colour Doppler to assess extrarenal vascular abnormalities or intrarenal changes.
- Use power Doppler to study vascular patterns in the cortex.

Box 12.6: Ultrasound images to record

- Sample spectral Doppler traces to record PSV and EDV of the suprarenal aorta, both renal arteries throughout their length, arteries at the renal hilum, and interlobar and interlobular vessels.

- Calculate AT and AI at the hilum and EDR and RI for intrarenal arteries.

- Spectral Doppler traces of both renal veins if a clinical indication is present.

- Spectral tracings at any sites of stenosis or occlusion, noting extent and location from the renal artery origin.

- Note features of atherosclerosis or fibromuscular dysplasia.

- B-mode to measure each kidney length (two to three measurements to calculate the average result).

- Power Doppler to show images of renal perfusion.

- Other pathology such as a renal cyst or calculus, or an abdominal aortic aneurysm.

13

COELIAC AND MESENTERIC ARTERIAL DISEASES

Atherosclerosis is not as common in these arteries as at other sites. Disease usually involves their origins and can be demonstrated by duplex scanning in more than 90 per cent of patients. There are non-atherosclerotic arterial diseases that have characteristic ultrasound features. Duplex scanning may be sufficient to detect disease, plan for interventional treatment and follow the results of treatment, but it is frequently used to select patients for other imaging techniques.

ANATOMY

Box 13.1: Arteries scanned for reporting

- Abdominal aorta
- Coeliac axis
- Splenic artery
- Hepatic arteries
- Left gastric artery
- Superior mesenteric artery: SMA
- Inferior mesenteric artery: IMA

The three main arterial branches of the abdominal aorta to the gastrointestinal track are the coeliac axis, SMA and IMA

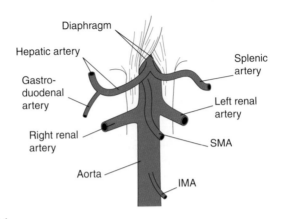

Fig. 13.1

The coeliac axis, SMA and IMA

- All arise from the anterior abdominal aorta.
- The coeliac axis is the first major branch of the abdominal aorta.
- The SMA origin is 1–2 cm distal to the coeliac axis and the IMA origin is 3–5 cm proximal to the aortic bifurcation.

(Figs 13.1–13.3). There are many potential connections between the three systems (Fig. 13.4).

Anatomical variations are common including:

- common or right hepatic artery from the SMA
- common hepatic artery from the aorta
- common trunk for the coeliac axis and SMA.

CLINICAL ASPECTS

Regional pathology, clinical presentations and treatment

Chronic mesenteric ischaemia

Stenosis or occlusion of the coeliac or mesenteric arteries or their branches can cause chronic intestinal ischaemia. The coeliac axis can be entrapped by the median arcuate ligament of the diaphragm. It usually requires two or all three arteries to be affected by high-grade

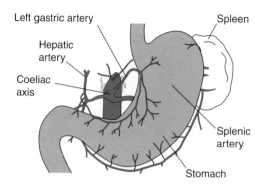

Fig. 13.2

The coeliac axis

- Divides into the common hepatic, splenic and left gastric arteries at 1–2 cm from its origin.
- The hepatic artery divides into right and left branches which enter the liver at the porta hepatis and lie adjacent to the right and left portal veins.
- The splenic artery is the largest, located superior and anterior to the splenic vein.
- The left gastric artery is the smallest.
- Supplies the liver, stomach and spleen.

Fig. 19.1 from Strandness DE. 1969: *Collateral Circulation in Clinical Surgery*. Philadelphia: WB Saunders. Reproduced with permission.

stenosis or occlusion to cause clinical symptoms, as there is rich collateral circulation.

Mesenteric ischaemia is considered in patients presenting with postprandial pain, weight loss and malabsorption, although these symptoms are usually due to other more common diseases. However, presentation can be with vague abdominal symptoms. Treatment is by surgical reconstruction or endovascular stenting.

Acute small bowel ischaemia

The SMA can be acutely occluded by an embolus from the heart. Acute thrombosis of the SMA or more distal small arteries and veins can occur, commonly due to severe dehydration, thrombophilia or as a complication of some therapeutic drugs. Presentation is usually

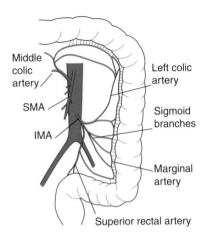

Fig. 13.3

The SMA and IMA

- The SMA lies to the left of the superior mesenteric vein, posterior to the splenic and portal veins and anterior to the left renal vein.
- The SMA origin is surrounded by an echogenic fat pad.
- The SMA supplies the distal duodenum, small intestine and proximal colon.
- The IMA supplies the distal colon and upper rectum.

Fig. 24.2 from Strandness DE. 1969: *Collateral Circulation in Clinical Surgery*. Philadelphia: WB Saunders. Reproduced with permission.

with abdominal pain, gastrointestinal bleeding, vomiting and diarrhoea or as profound shock. Treatment is usually by surgical reconstruction or resection of infarcted bowel.

Visceral artery aneurysms

Visceral aneurysms are uncommon but can occur in the splenic or hepatic arteries or SMA. They are detected incidentally by ultrasound or from wall calcification seen with plain X-ray, and are asymptomatic until they present with rupture that is usually intraperitoneal and catastrophic. Treatment is by ligation or excision and bypass grafting. Ultrasound can distinguish an aneurysm from an abdominal cyst.

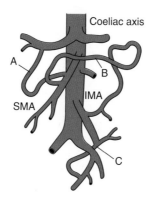

Fig. 13.4

Collaterals between the three main visceral arteries

A: Coeliac axis to the SMA through the gastroduodenal and pancreaticoduodenal arteries.

B: Middle colic branch of the SMA to the left colic branch of the IMA – the 'meandering mesenteric artery'.

C: Left colic branch of the IMA to rectal branches of the internal iliac artery – the 'marginal artery of Drummond'.

Differential diagnosis

Chronic or acute abdominal pain is more likely to result from

- appendicitis
- cholecystitis
- pancreatitis
- peptic ulceration
- renal colic
- leaking or ruptured abdominal aortic aneurysm.

What the doctors need to know

- Is there stenosis in the coelic axis, SMA or IMA and how severe is it?
- Is there evidence of extrinsic compression of the coeliac axis origin?
- Is there occlusion of one or more of the arteries or their branches?
- Is there an aneurysm of one of the arteries, where is it and what is its diameter?

- What is the flow direction in arteries that may act as collaterals with stenosis or occlusion of the coeliac axis or SMA?
- Are there anatomical variations?

THE DUPLEX SCAN

Normal arterial flow

Coeliac axis

The axis and its major branches show similar low-resistance flow patterns with a sharp systolic upstroke consistent with flow into the liver and spleen and PSV <200 cm/s (Fig. 13.5). Taking food does not affect flow. The gastric artery is rarely seen with ultrasound. The splenic artery may show turbulent flow due to tortuosity.

SMA

The flow pattern varies according to the metabolic activity of the intestine (Fig. 13.6). In the fasting state, the SMA normally exhibits a high-resistance pattern with a sharp systolic upstroke and variable diastolic component with low forward flow, reversed flow or both. The PSV is < 275 cm/s and is usually between 100 and 140 cm/s. After ingesting a meal, there is normally a considerable increase in SMA blood flow over 20–30 min, a fall in resistance, a three fold increase in EDV and an increase in arterial diameter.

Anatomical variations

If there is a common trunk for the coeliac axis and SMA then there will be a low-resistance signal at the origin changing to a high-resistance signal in the SMA distal to the origins of the hepatic and splenic arteries. A low-resistance signal will also be present in the proximal SMA if the common or right hepatic artery arises from it more distally.

IMA

If seen, the waveform is similar to the SMA with a high-resistance pattern but less reversed diastolic flow. Normal and abnormal values for PSVs have not been defined but velocities are not as high as in the SMA. IMA velocities are not likely to be affected by ingesting food.

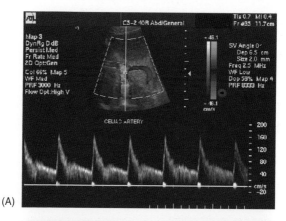

Fig. 13.5

Normal coeliac axis

A: Spectral Doppler.
B: Colour Doppler.

Note the bifurcation forming the hepatic and splenic arteries to produce the 'seagull sign'.

Indications for scanning

Symptoms and signs that may lead to a scan are:

- abdominal pain
- non-specific weight loss

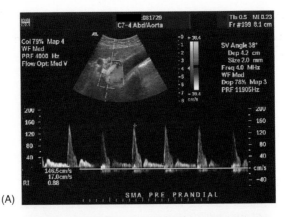

(A)

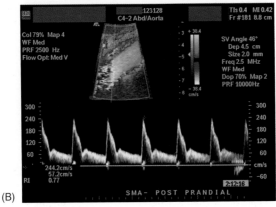

(B)

Fig. 13.6

Spectral analysis for SMA waveforms with:

A: a high-resistance signal in the fasting state

B: increased velocities with high diastolic velocities and absence of reverse flow after a standard meal.

- malabsorption
- epigastric bruit.

Visceral arteries may need to be scanned to:

- screen for mesenteric ischaemia
- demonstrate coeliac axis compression by the median arcuate ligament

Table 13.1 Criteria for coeliac artery stenosis

Stenosis	PSV (cm/s)	EDV (cm/s)	Post-stenotic turbulence
50–70%	>200	>45	Present
Severe	>300	>100	Severe

- detect a visceral artery aneurysm
- monitor known arterial stenosis
- follow up after intervention for stenotic disease.

Criteria for diagnosing disease

Criteria recommended are based on studies by Moneta, and by Zwolak and colleagues. (Moneta GL. Screening for mesenteric vascular insufficiency and follow-up of mesenteric artery bypass procedures. *Seminars in Vascular Surgery* 2001;**14**:186–192. Zwolak RM, Fillinger MF, Walsh DB *et al.* Mesenteric and celiac duplex scanning: a validation study. *Journal of Vascular Surgery* 1998; **27**:1078–1087.)

Coeliac artery stenosis or occlusion

Criteria for coeliac artery stenosis are shown in Table 13.1.

Stenosis or occlusion usually affects the first 1–2 cm of the artery (Fig. 13.7). Occlusion is associated with absent colour Doppler image and loss of spectral signal. Retrograde flow in the hepatic artery is diagnostic for severe coeliac artery stenosis or occlusion. It is helpful to evaluate the hepatic artery if the coeliac axis is difficult to identify or at an angle that makes it difficult to obtain accurate Doppler samples.

Coeliac axis stenosis due to median arcuate ligament compression causes high PSVs during normal respiration that disappear with deep inspiration or by making the patient stand. The origin appears to be 'bent' upwards losing its straight orientation.

SMA stenosis or occlusion

Criteria for SMA stenosis are shown in Table 13.2.

Stenosis or occlusion usually affects the proximal artery. Occlusion is associated with absent colour Doppler image and loss of the spectral

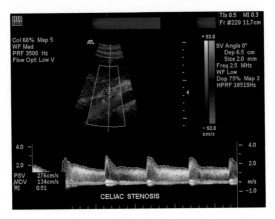

Fig. 13.7

Spectral tracing for severe coeliac artery stenosis

Table 13.2 Criteria for SMA stenosis

Stenosis	PSV (cm/s)	EDV (cm/s)	Post-stenotic turbulence
50–70%	>275	>45	Present
Severe	>350	>100	Severe

signal in the SMA. Retrograde flow may be seen in the first set of branches of the SMA feeding the more distal artery.

For SMA stenosis:

- post-prandial studies add little to the examination if the fasting PSV is raised, and should only be performed if there is post-prandial pain
- the decrease in PSV beyond an SMA stenosis or occlusion is less if there is a good collateral circulation feeding the SMA
- a low-resistance Doppler signal in the IMA, or B-mode evidence of dilatation suggest it is acting as a collateral for occlusive disease in the SMA or coeliac axis.

PROTOCOLS FOR SCANNING

Follow the principles for abdominal scanning discussed on page 43 in Chapter 2.

Prepare the patient

The patient fasts with the scan ideally performed in the morning. There must be access to the abdomen from the sternum to well below the umbilicus. If a post-prandial study is requested, give the patient a high-calorie, high-protein drink (flavoured milk) and biscuits, and repeat scanning after 20 min. Ask the patient to be prepared to hold the breath to capture a signal.

Select the best transducer

Use a low-frequency curved array transducer. A phased array transducer may be preferred to angle upwards beneath the xiphoid process or in the intercostal spaces.

Aorta, coeliac axis and mesenteric arteries

Position the patient and select a window

Lay the patient supine on the table, image through an anterior window, and move to a left lateral decubitus position or tilt the patient to slight reverse Trendelenburg if bowel gas is a problem.

Scanning techniques

- Identify the suprarenal aorta and obtain an aortic PSV above the level of the coeliac axis.
- Examine for aortic aneurysm or other disease if present (see Chapter 8).
- Use colour Doppler to examine the length of the coeliac axis, the SMA and IMA to detect localized flow abnormalities. Use B-mode to visualize plaque. 'Walk' the Doppler sample throughout all arteries to ensure that a focal increase in PSV is not missed. Adjust the sample volume to be slightly less than the arterial diameter. Determine the flow direction in branches.
- Identify the coeliac artery and measure PSV and EDV at the origin, proximal trunk and bifurcation into hepatic and splenic arteries.
- Identify the SMA distal to the coeliac origin arising from the anterior aorta. It is usually possible to follow the artery out for 5 cm. Measure PSV and EDV at the origin, proximal and distal SMA.

- Note whether the IMA is patent, occluded or not visualized. The IMA is more frequently seen in longitudinal rather than transverse. If found in transverse then it is at about 12–2 o'clock from the aorta. The IMA may not be detected unless it is acting as a collateral with occlusive disease of the coeliac axis or SMA, or if the patient is thin.
- Perform a limited examination of the hepatoportal venous circulation (see page 297 in Chapter 14).

Pitfalls!

- Because of anatomical variations, do not assume an artery is occluded if it is not seen.
- Tortuosity of the coeliac axis can make if difficult to obtain an accurate angle of insonation.
- Calcification can cause shadowing that may be incorrectly interpreted as an occlusion.
- Increased flow in a mesenteric artery as a compensatory mechanism can be incorrectly interpreted as being due to stenosis – always determine whether or not there is post-stenotic turbulence.
- A collateral adjacent to an occluded artery can be incorrectly interpreted as the normal artery.

Box 13.2: Ultrasound images to record

- Sample spectral Doppler traces to record PSV and EDV of the arteries listed in Box 13.1.
- Spectral Doppler traces of the SMA post-prandial if requested.
- Spectral tracings at any sites of stenosis or occlusion, noting the extent and location from the artery origin.
- Other pathology such as portal venous pathology or an abdominal aortic aneurysm.

14

HEPATOPORTAL VENOUS DISEASES

Intrinsic vascular disease or extrinsic vascular compression can cause obstruction of the extra- or intrahepatic portal or hepatic venous systems. Ultrasound is used to assess vascular changes that result from portal hypertension, plan for interventional treatment, and perform surveillance after intervention.

ANATOMY

Box 14.1: Vessels scanned for reporting

- Portal vein
- Hepatic veins
- Splenic vein
- Superior mesenteric vein: SMV
- Left gastric (coronary) vein
- Hepatic artery
- Superior mesenteric artery: SMA
- Inferior mesenteric vein: IMV
- Inferior vena cava: IVC

Abdominal veins drain to the IVC or portal venous systems (Fig. 14.1).

There may be congenital abnormality of the infrarenal IVC (Fig. 14.2).

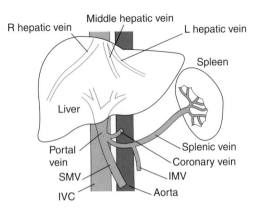

Fig. 14.1

Systemic, portal and hepatic veins

- The SMV and splenic vein join to form the portal vein.
- The portal vein is anterior to the IVC and SMA.
- The portal vein divides into right and left branches at the porta hepatis to accompany hepatic artery branches into the liver.
- Major anatomical variations of the portal vein are uncommon but include agenesis of the right or left portal vein, trifurcation at the porta hepatis, a right anterior portal branch arising from the left portal vein, or a right posterior portal branch arising from the main portal vein.
- Three main hepatic veins pass from the back of liver to the IVC immediately below the diaphragm.

Portosystemic collaterals

Several sites for anastomosis between portal and systemic veins can develop as collaterals or varices if the hepatoportal venous circulation is compromised (Fig. 14.3).

- **The left gastric (coronary) vein** joins the junction of the SMV and portal vein and connects to the systemic oesophageal veins at the gastro-oesophageal junction and to veins around the left lobe of liver.
- **The paraumbilical vein** joins the left branch of the portal vein and passes through the ligamentum teres to connect with systemic veins of the abdominal wall at the umbilicus.
- **Spleno-systemic collaterals** pass to the pancreatic head or gastro-oesophageal region.

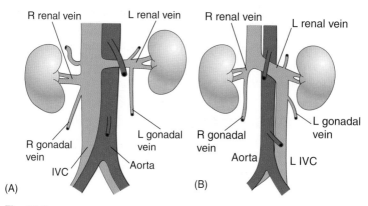

Fig. 14.2

IVC

A: Normal anatomy.

B: Anomalous left-sided IVC from persistence of the embryological azygos vein.

Fig. 23.14 from Zwiebel WJ. 1994: *Introduction to Vascular Ultrasonography*. Philadelphia: WB Saunders. Reproduced with permission.

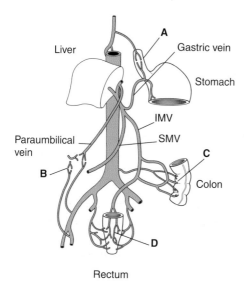

Fig. 14.3

Potential sites for anastomosis between portal and systemic venous tributaries.

A: Oesophagus
B: Umbilicus
C: Colon
D: Rectum

- Spleno-renal collaterals connect with the left renal and gonadal veins.
- IMV tributaries connect with veins draining to the internal iliac veins at the colon and rectum.
- Retroperitoneal varices can form a 'tumour-like' mass.

CLINICAL ASPECTS

Duplex scanning is performed in patients with clinical features of chronic hepatic or splenic disease. Other investigations that may be required are endoscopy, transjugular measurement of the hepatic venous pressure gradient, liver biopsy, computed tomography, magnetic resonance imaging and angiography.

Regional pathology
Portal hypertension

Portal hypertension is elevated pressure in the portal venous system due to increased resistance to flow and splanchnic vasodilatation. Flow is diverted to systemic veins through collaterals. In the late phase, a thrombosed portal vein becomes small and is replaced by collaterals or a cavernous venous malformation at the porta hepatis.

Portal hypertension is classified as:

- prehepatic:
  - portal or splenic vein thrombosis from cirrhosis, coagulation disorders, malignancy, intra-abdominal sepsis or from unknown causes
  - portal or splenic vein obstruction from pancreatitis, pancreatic carcinoma or hepatocellular carcinoma
- intrahepatic:
  - alcoholic cirrhosis
  - post-hepatitis cirrhosis
  - idiopathic non-cirrhotic portal fibrosis
- posthepatic (Budd–Chiari syndrome):
  - hepatic venous or IVC thrombosis – veno-occlusive disease
  - extrinsic compression by tumours
  - IVC web, mostly in Asians.

The Budd–Chiari syndrome

The syndrome consists of hepatosplenomegaly, ascites and upper abdominal pain due to thrombosis or occlusion in intrahepatic venules, hepatic veins or suprahepatic IVC. Not all hepatic veins are necessarily involved. It is caused by myeloproliferative disorders, thrombophilia, a congenital web in the IVC, extrinsic compression by a large caudate lobe or hepatic tumour, or from unknown aetiology. There is congestive liver damage, the severity of which is determined by the extent of thrombosis and development of venous collaterals. Portal hypertension can cause gastrointestinal bleeding, and cirrhosis may later be complicated by hepatocellular carcinoma.

Clinical presentations

Gastrointestinal haemorrhage

This can result from increased pressure in portosystemic collaterals, particularly with bleeding from submucosal varices in the lower oesophagus or cardia and fundus of the stomach. Haemorrhage from varices occurs in some 50 per cent of patients with cirrhosis, and has an immediate mortality rate of >10 per cent. There is an approximate 50 per cent risk of rebleeding and 50 per cent mortality within 1–2 years without treatment. The incidence of haemorrhage is high if flow in collaterals is towards the SVC and low if flow is towards the IVC. There is splenomegaly and anaemia due to hypersplenism in approximately 50 per cent.

Ascites

Ascites is most often secondary to cirrhosis. It is usually a relatively early presentation and may be precipitated by fluid retention, heart failure or intraperitoneal malignancy.

Hepatic encephalopathy

The liver normally detoxifies products from the digestive tract, and diversion of flow by portosystemic shunting can lead to hepatic encephalopathy. Breakdown products of protein metabolism are particularly toxic. Potentially reversible neurological deficit is caused by shunting blood from the portal to systemic circulation, either through collaterals or a surgical connection. Spontaneous development has an insidious onset with intellectual deterioration, and advanced stages can lead to coma.

Hepatorenal syndrome

This is a severe complication of advanced liver disease with portal hypertension and ascites. It can be precipitated by shock, infection, surgery, large-volume paracentesis or nephrotoxic drugs. It results from intense splanchnic vasodilatation causing reduced effective blood volume, leading to renal vasoconstriction. The process is reversible with treatment.

Endocrine dysfunction

Hypothyroidism, and feminization and hypogonadism in males are features of liver disease and result from failure to metabolize pituitary hormones.

Coagulation disorders

Increased risk of bleeding in liver disease results from failure to synthesize coagulation factors.

Treatment

Medical measures are the first line of treatment in all patients. If intervention is required to treat complications, this can be by:

- portosystemic shunting
- transjugular intrahepatic portosystemic shunting (TIPS)
- liver transplantation.

Portosystemic shunting

This has been the traditional technique to decompress the portal venous circulation. The object is to prevent recurrence of haemorrhage from varices. However, it is a major operation with appreciable mortality, it can cause encephalopathy and interfere with the ability to use the vessels to anastomose for liver transplantation. Various techniques are available (Fig. 14.4). The portal vein, SMV or splenic vein is anastomosed to the IVC or a major tributary such as the left renal vein.

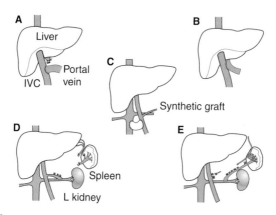

Fig. 14.4

Portosystemic shunts

A: End-to-side anastomosis of the portal vein to the IVC to divert all portal blood into the systemic circulation.

B: Side-to-side anastomosis of the portal vein to the IVC to divert some flow but partially preserve portal flow to the liver.

C: Synthetic bypass from the portal vein to the IVC if the veins cannot be brought together.

D: End-to-side anastomosis of the proximal splenic vein to the left renal vein so as to preserve the portal vein.

E: End-to-side anastomosis of the distal splenic vein to the left renal vein.

Fig. 101-4 from Terblanche J, in Rutherford RB (ed). 1995: *Vascular Surgery*. Philadelphia: WB Saunders. Reproduced with permission.

Percutaneous transjugular intrahepatic portosystemic shunting (TIPS)

This has largely replaced surgical shunting, with percutaneous insertion of a stent between a large branch of the hepatic and portal venous systems, usually to the right portal vein (Fig. 14.5). TIPS is equivalent to side-to-side portocaval shunting. It does not interfere with the subsequent ability to perform liver transplantation. It can be complicated by hepatic encephalopathy. TIPS may be the definitive treatment for portal hypertension but it has a high restenosis rate. Alternatively, TIPS may be used as a temporary measure while waiting for transplantation. The procedure is usually performed under fluoroscopic control but ultrasound has been used to select the most

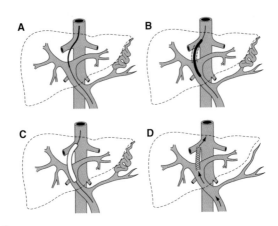

Fig. 14.5

The technique for TIPS

A: Percutaneous puncture to thread a needle-tipped guide-wire through the internal jugular vein to the IVC, and through a hepatic vein to a portal vein branch.

B: A balloon threaded over the wire is expanded to form a track between the two circulations and is then removed.

C: A stent is then threaded over the wire and deployed in the track.

D: The deployed stent maintains a channel between the two circulations.

Fig. 101-3 from Terblanche J, in Rutherford RB (ed). 1995: *Vascular Surgery*. Philadelphia: WB Saunders. Reproduced with permission.

suitable veins and guide the needle used to establish the connection. Liver function may improve and hepatic haemodynamics may return towards normal after TIPS due to hypertrophy of remaining non-cirrhotic liver tissue.

Transplantation

Transplantation has become widely accepted as the definitive treatment for advanced liver disease as immunosuppression techniques have become more effective.

Selection of treatment

Active bleeding can be controlled by pharmacological agents that cause venoconstriction and by balloon tamponade. Endoscopic techniques are then used to sclerose or ligate varices. Primary bleeding is not usually an indication for prophylaxis by operative intervention.

Indications for portosystemic shunting or TIPS are:

● intractable variceal haemorrhage
● recurrent variceal bleeding after failure of endoscopic treatment
● refractory ascites
● Budd–Chiari syndrome and veno-occlusive disease.

Contraindications to shunting or TIPS are progressive liver failure, pulmonary hypertension and severe hepatic encephalopathy.

Liver transplantation may be required for liver failure from cirrhosis due to hepatitis C, alcohol-related cirrhosis, portal or hepatic vein thrombosis, biliary atresia, refractory ascites, the hepatorenal syndrome or malignancy.

What the doctors need to know

● Is there patency and flow in the portal vein and its tributaries?
● Is there patency and flow in the hepatic veins and IVC?
● Are collateral veins and portosystemic venous connections present?
● Are venous connections or vascular anastomoses patent after portosystemic shunting, TIPS or liver transplantation, and what is their size?
● What is the state of the biliary tree?
● What are the sizes and composition of the liver, spleen and pancreas?
● Is ascites present?

THE DUPLEX SCAN

Normal findings
Portal and hepatic venous flow

● Normal portal venous flow is always towards the liver (**hepatopetal**). Flow in the hepatic artery and branches is in the same direction and it can be difficult to distinguish between them

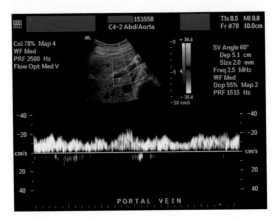

Fig. 14.6

Normal spectral tracing from a portal vein

with colour Doppler. Portal venous flow away from the liver (**hepatofugal**) always indicates disease.

● The portal venous waveform shows continuous flow, with an average velocity of 15–20 cm/s, that is not pulsatile but is phasic with respiration such that flow tends to fall during inspiration and rise during expiration (Fig. 14.6).

● Colour Doppler should fill the lumen of all veins.

● The portal vein diameter measured where it crosses the IVC is <13 mm with quiet respiration increasing to <16 mm with deep inspiration.

● SMV and splenic vein diameters increase by 20–100 per cent during inspiration and decrease with expiration.

● Portal vein and SMV flow and diameters increase after a meal, while flow falls after exercise.

● Hepatic veins show triphasic flow reflecting the right heart signal as well as respiratory fluctuations (Fig. 14.7).

● It should be possible to identify three patent hepatic veins.

Normal findings after intervention

Portosystemic shunting

Normal patency is confirmed by demonstrating:

● flow through the anastomosis from the portal to systemic circulation shown by colour and spectral Doppler

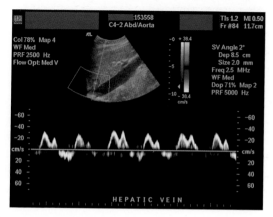

Fig. 14.7

Normal spectral tracing from an hepatic vein

- dilatation of the IVC or other recipient vein
- reduced size and number of collaterals
- phasic flow with respiration in portal vein tributaries
- hepatofugal flow in intrahepatic portal veins if there is side-to-side portocaval shunt, reduced ascites and splenomegaly.

TIPS

Normal patency is shown by:

- hepatopetal flow in the main portal vein
- maximum portal venous velocity of double normal values to 30–40 cm/s with spectral broadening from turbulence, and respiratory and cardiac fluctuations of flow
- hepatic artery velocity increased by >50 per cent
- decrease in the number and size of collaterals
- reduced ascites and splenomegaly.

Indications for scanning

Clinical presentations

Symptoms, signs and complications that may lead to a scan are:

- abdominal pain
- ascites

- hepatosplenomegaly
- symptoms of liver failure
- gastrointestinal bleeding
- pancreatic disease.

Selection for intervention

Duplex scanning is used to help select suitable patients prior to portosystemic shunting, TIPS or liver transplantation. Examine for normal anatomy of the portal vein, hepatic veins, IVC, hepatic artery and biliary system. Note hepatic tumours or other diseases. If there is any uncertainty then investigation is likely to proceed to angiography or other imaging techniques.

Surveillance after intervention

The very high incidence of stent stenosis or occlusion in the stent after TIPS makes post-operative surveillance essential, with duplex scanning recommended at 48 hours, every three months for the first year and then six-monthly. Stenosis at the anastomosis after shunting or transplantation will result in reversion to features of portal hypertension.

Criteria for diagnosing disease

Portal hypertension

Ultrasound findings with portal hypertension include:

- to-and-fro (biphasic) portal venous flow with moderate disease, and hepatofugal flow in approximately 5 per cent with severe disease – this is **diagnostic**
- presence of portosystemic collaterals or varices – these are **highly specific**
- demonstration of a recanalized paraumbilical vein $\geqslant 3$ mm diameter with hepatofugal flow in the ligamentum teres, a **highly specific and sensitive** sign for intra- or posthepatic portal hypertension
- enlarged portal vein >13 mm with inspiration – present in approximately 50 per cent and **highly specific**
- enlarged left gastric vein and coronary vein >6–7 mm diameter

- decreased portal vein flow velocity – this is **highly variable**
  <20 per cent increase in splenic vein or SMV diameter with change from quiet respiration to deep inspiration – **specific and sensitive** but difficult in practice
- thready hepatic veins that are difficult to sample
- abnormal liver texture
- splenomegaly (coronal length >13 cm) in 50 per cent
- ascites.

Portal vein thrombosis

This is associated with:

- enlarged portal vein filled with thrombus if acute
- small, echogenic portal vein if there is chronic occlusion, often difficult to distinguish from liver parenchyma
- no evidence of venous flow in the portal vein or at the porta hepatis when Doppler sensitivity has been maximized
- cavernous transformation of the portal vein with tortuous collaterals at the porta hepatis – these demonstrate the same flow pattern as the now thrombosed portal vein
- numerous large varices representing portosystemic shunts with continuous low-velocity portal venous flow
- a coronary vein diameter >6–7 mm
- increased hepatic arterial flow.

Budd–Chiari syndrome

Ultrasound features from the hepatic veins are:

- no colour or spectral flow signal if thrombosed, or otherwise
- reversed, turbulent, or monophasic flow
- thickened vein wall and vein dilatation
- intrahepatic collaterals
- abnormal vein course
- extrahepatic anastomoses.

Ultrasound features in the portal venous system are as previously described. Ultrasound features in the IVC are abnormal or there is absent flow, and thrombosis, stenosis or membrane.

Liver disease

B-mode can be used to distinguish diffuse liver disease due to cirrhosis (nodular liver surface and texture), non-cirrhotic portal fibrosis (diffuse texture), or fatty infiltration (increased parenchymal echogenicity) with moderate accuracy. Increasing degrees of fatty infiltration are associated with increasing difficulty in visualizing intrahepatic vessels. B-mode also detects liver tumours, and colour Doppler is used to assess their vascularity. Ultrasound guidance can be used for transjugular or percutaneous biopsy. Ultrasound provides additional information about liver, biliary, splenic or pancreatic disease.

Splanchnic haemodynamics differ for chronic liver diseases and haematological diseases causing splenomegaly. Splenomegaly due to cirrhosis causes decreased portal flow velocity, increased splenic artery resistance and large oesophageal varices, whereas these findings are not observed with primary splenomegaly.

Portosystemic shunting

Criteria that indicate anastomotic stenosis have not been defined, but any increase above the normal maximum flow velocity of 40 cm/s is likely to lead to further investigation.

TIPS

- Stent stenosis will cause the maximum velocity to fall to <90–100 cm/s in the portal vein and to rise to >190–200 cm/s in the stent.
- Stent occlusion results in absent flow within the stent and to either side.
- There may be a change from hepatofugal to hepatopetal flow in the left portal vein.

Liver transplantation

After transplantation, ultrasound is used to detect:

- occlusion of the anastomosed hepatic artery or portal vein, or IVC thrombosis
- liver infarction

- pseudoaneurysm
- obstructed draining bile ducts
- allograft rejection: unlike kidney transplants, rejection of liver transplants is not associated with increased hepatic artery resistance.

Criteria that indicate anastomotic stenosis have not been defined but any increase in portal venous or hepatic arterial flow velocities at the anastomoses is likely to lead to further investigation.

PROTOCOLS FOR SCANNING

Follow the general principles for abdominal scanning discussed on page 43 in Chapter 2.

Prepare the patient

The patient fasts with the scan ideally performed in the morning (see page 50 in Chapter 3). There must be access to the upper abdomen. Ask the patient to be prepared to hold the breath to capture an image.

Select the best transducer

Use a low-frequency curved array transducer. The phased array transducer may be preferred to angle upwards beneath the xiphoid process or in the intercostal spaces. A higher-frequency transducer is required to show a recanalized paraumbilical vein.

Hepatoportal veins

Position the patient and select a window

Lay the patient supine on the table. If the scan is difficult, move to a left lateral decubitus position with the liver as a window, or tilt the patient to slight reverse Trendelenburg to allow the viscera to descend if bowel gas is a problem. The patient may need to be booked for prior abdominal paracentesis if there is marked ascites. Suitable windows include:

- a right subcostal or intercostal window for the portal veins
- a left intercostal axillary view through the spleen for the distal splenic vein

- right subcostal, intercostal and xiphisternum windows viewed in transverse for hepatic veins
- a right intercostal window with the patient in left lateral decubitus for the right hepatic vein or TIPS stent.

Use settings for low flow states (see Chapter 2).

Scanning techniques for the portal vein and its tributaries

- Examine the veins in B-mode and colour Doppler. Determine patency and flow direction, and obtain spectral signals and diameters for each vein.
- Identify the splenic vein near the midline and follow it to the left as it passes transverse then deeper and cephalad to the hilum of the spleen.
- Trace the splenic vein to the right, to its junction with the portal vein so as to distinguish the portal vein from the IVC and bile ducts.
- Follow the portal vein cephalad to its division into right and left portal veins near the porta hepatis.
- Then follow the portal vein caudally and medial to its origin.
- View the SMV in longitudinal from its confluence with the splenic vein and take spectral signals to distinguish it from the SMA.
- Examine the liver texture and surface. Record the coronal length of the spleen and presence of ascites.
- Perform a limited examination of the splanchnic arterial circulation.
- If no flow seen in the portal vein, maximize Doppler sensitivity by using a low Doppler scale, low wall filter, minimal angle of insonation to direction of flow, and a high-frequency transducer.

Scanning techniques for the hepatic veins

- Examine the veins in B-mode and colour Doppler. Determine patency and flow direction, and obtain spectral signals and diameters for each vein.
- Scan more cephalad to examine each hepatic vein as it passes to the IVC near the right atrium.
- Use colour Doppler as they can be difficult to identify with B-mode alone particularly if there is extrinsic compression.

Box 14.2: Differentiation of portal and hepatic veins in the liver

These are seen as echolucent structures. They can be differentiated with ultrasound.

● Portal veins are surrounded by a dense fibrous sheath.
● Portal veins are larger at the porta hepatis and hepatic veins enlarge as they pass towards the IVC.
● Portal veins converge at the porta hepatis and hepatic veins converge as they pass towards the IVC.
● The intrahepatic branches of the portal veins tend to run transversely and hepatic veins tend to run vertically.
● Portal venous flow is phasic with respiration while hepatic venous flow is phasic but also reflects right atrial pulsations.

Collateral veins

● Search for collaterals at the splenic hilum, in the midline, at the gall bladder fossa, along the surface of the liver, and at the anterior abdominal wall.
● Examine collaterals in B-mode and colour Doppler. Obtain spectral signals to indicate their presence and flow direction, and measure diameters for each vein.
● Scan in longitudinal for the coronary vein extending cephalad from the SMV near its confluence with the portal vein.
● The ligamentum teres runs obliquely to the left and is seen as an echogenic band with a hypoechoic channel. Its location is variable. Scan for the paraumbilical vein in the ligamentum teres looking for the presence and direction of flow, and measure the diameter of the hypoechoic lumen.

Portosystemic shunt or liver transplant

Perform a hepatoportal venous and hepatic arterial study as described above and note patency and record maximum velocities at anastomosis sites.

TIPS

The stent is easily seen in the liver as a highly echogenic but non-shadowing structure usually connecting a hepatic vein deep in the right lobe and a branch of the portal vein at the porta hepatis.

Note patency and flow direction, and record velocities from:

● multiple sites in the stent and adjacent veins
● other intrahepatic veins if the stent cannot be clearly seen due to bowel gas
● the right and left portal veins
● the extrahepatic portal vein
● the SMV and splenic vein at their confluence
● all main hepatic veins
● the IVC.

Identify the stent in B-mode in longitudinal, oblique and transverse and note its location and extension into the hepatic and portal veins to detect stent migration with serial scans.

Box 14.3: Ultrasound images to record

● Sample spectral Doppler traces to record flow direction in vessels listed in Box 14.1 and in the stent for TIPS or anastomoses for portosystemic shunts and transplants.
● Spectral traces of the hepatic arteries at any sites of stenosis or occlusion, noting the extent and location from the vessel origin.
● Colour Doppler to show the presence of collaterals and spectral Doppler to show flow directions.
● B-mode of the diameters of hepatoportal veins and collaterals.
● Colour and spectral Doppler to show thrombosis of portal or hepatic veins.
● B-mode assessment of the texture and surface of the liver and size of the spleen.
● Other pathology such as ascites or hepatic cyst or tumour.

15

PENILE VASCULAR DISEASES

Duplex scanning is part of the diagnostic process in most services that study erectile dysfunction in males because it is relatively atraumatic and inexpensive. It helps to establish the cause so as to better choose appropriate treatment. However, there is now a tendency to consider that the trauma and expense of investigation is not warranted because of the introduction of sildenafil citrate (Viagra) which is increasingly used to treat all causes.

ANATOMY

Box 15.1: Vessels scanned for reporting

- Aorta
- Common iliac artery: CIA
- Internal iliac artery: IIA
- Penile artery
- Cavernosal artery

Other vessels discussed

- Internal pudendal artery
- Bulbo-urethral artery
- Dorsal artery

Erectile tissue is in the corpora cavernosa and corpus spongiosum (Fig. 15.1).

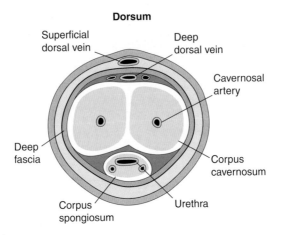

Fig. 15.1

Cross-section of the penis

- The corpora cavernosa form the main part of the body and are located dorso-laterally separated by a median septum.
- The corpus spongiosum surrounds the urethra.
- They are ensheathed by the deep fascia (tunica albuginea).

Redrawn from Fig. P31 of Scott R. 1982: *Urology Illustrated.* ©1982, with permission from Elsevier.

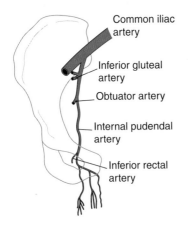

Fig.15.2

The internal iliac circulation in the male

The terminal branch to the penis is the internal pudendal artery which continues as the penile artery.

Fig. 13.4 from Queral L, in: Bergan JJ and Yao JS. 1979: *Surgery of the Aorta and its Body Branches.* New York: Grune and Stratton. Reproduced with permission.

The arterial supply to the penis is from the internal iliac circulation (Fig. 15.2) through the paired internal pudendal arteries becoming the penile arteries (Fig. 15.3). The venous drainage is mostly from a dorsal vein of the penis to the internal pudendal vein to return to the internal iliac vein.

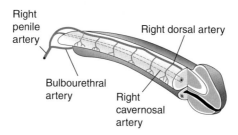

Fig. 15.3

Penile artery branches

- The bulbourethral artery supplies the corpus spongiosurn and urethra.
- Paired dorsal arteries supply the skin and glans penis.
- Paired cavernosal arteries give small branches termed helicine arterioles that progressively divide to form lacunae in each corpus cavernosum.

Redrawn from Fig. P31 of Scott R. 1982: *Urology Illustrated*. ©1982, with permission from Elsevier.

CLINICAL ASPECTS

Regional pathology

Erectile dysfunction (impotence)

Normal erection is a neurovascular phenomenon. Somatosensory afferents from the penis excite centres in the hind brain and spinal cord. Sympathetic and parasympathetic autonomic efferent nerves then induce a vascular response. There is smooth muscle relaxation of cavernous arterioles resulting in vasodilatation and increased arterial inflow relative to venous outflow. Distension of sinusoids causes mechanical compression of draining venules against the tunica albuginea preventing venous outflow.

Erectile dysfunction has various causes including:

- **arterial insufficiency** due to:
  - aortic occlusion causing the Leriche syndrome (see page 146 in Chapter 8)
  - CIA or IIA stenosis
  - diffuse internal pudendal or penile artery stenosis or occlusion
- **venous leakage** due to:
  - insufficient corporal veno-occlusion.
  - leakage through enlarged veins

- cavernosal disorders:
  - inability of venous channels to enlarge due to Peyronie's disease
  - inability of cavernous smooth muscle to relax due to fibrosis
  - abnormal communications between the corpora cavernosa and spongiosum
- neurological damage from:
  - spinal cord injury
  - surgical pelvic dissection, for example during repair of an abdominal aortic aneurysm
  - sympathetic nerve block or sympathectomy
  - autonomic nerve disorders
- psychogenic disorders.

Vasculogenic dysfunction is frequently mixed arterial and venous. It is more common in association with diabetes, smoking and excessive alcohol consumption. Other risk factors for arterial disease are hypertension and hypercholesterolaemia.

Mechanical disorders

Peyronie's disease is an uncommon condition of unknown aetiology. It may be caused by repeated minor trauma and is frequently associated with Dupuytren's contracture of the hands. Normal elastic tissue of the tunica is replaced by scar tissue, usually on the dorsum leading to upward curvature during erection. Many patients have abnormal arterial studies.

High-flow priapism is persisting erection following trauma to the penis or perineum causing injury to an artery with high flow through a fistula into the corpora cavernosa.

Low-flow priapism is persisting erection associated with decreased outflow, most often due to injection of vasoactive drugs to test for erectile dysfunction.

Clinical assessment

It is necessary to obtain a medical history for diabetes, hypertension, heart disease and hypercholesterolaemia, alcohol ingestion, and smoking, and a sexual and psychiatric history. The penis is examined for physical deformities or tumours.

Treatment

In the past, there were many options including:

- penile intracavernosal injection of vasoactive drugs
- a penile prosthesis
- arterial revascularization
- surgery to ligate leaking veins.

Most patients are now treated with Viagra.

What the doctors need to know

- Is there reduced arterial inflow?
- Is there venous leakage?
- Is there a cavernosal abnormality such as Peyronie's disease?
- Is there no vascular abnormality suggesting a psychological or neurological cause?

THE DUPLEX SCAN

Box 15.2: Abbreviations
- PSV: peak systolic velocity
- EDV: end diastolic velocity
- AT: acceleration time = time from onset to the first peak in systole
- RI: resistance index = $(1 - EDV/PSV)$

Normal findings

Normal function has been studied by duplex scanning in volunteers with a flaccid penis and then after erection is induced by giving a vasoactive drug including:

- intracorporeal papaverine
- intraurethral papaverine
- intracorporeal prostaglandin E
- oral Viagra.

These may be supplemented by visual or physical stimulation.

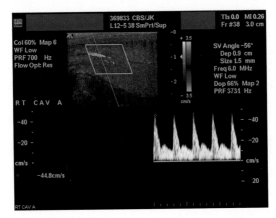

Fig. 15.4

Normal spectral Doppler trace from a cavernosal artery in the flaccid penis.

Injection techniques are commonly used although the simplicity of oral Viagra appeals to many, particularly since intracorporeal drugs occasionally cause low-flow priapism. It is necessary to wait for 30–45 min after oral Viagra to obtain maximum effect.

While the penis is **flaccid**:

● it is not possible to detect the helicine arterioles even with power Doppler
● there is low-resistance forward systolic and diastolic flow
● the PSV in the cavernosal artery is >40 cm/s (Fig. 15.4)
● the AT is <75 ms
● the EDV is 5–10 cm/s due to low intracavernosal resistance.

During **erection**:

● flow becomes apparent in the cavernosal arteries and helicine arterioles
● there are progressive changes in diastolic flow:
  ● in the early phase, there is prominent diastolic flow due to decreased resistance
  ● end diastolic flow is then lost as intracavernosal pressure rises

- reverse end diastolic flow is then seen as intracavernosal pressure exceeds the diastolic pressure
- diastolic flow is lost when the penis becomes rigid
- there is increased PSV >80 cm/s in the proximal cavernosal arteries
- the cavernosal artery demonstrates a >70 per cent increase in diameter
- there is increased venous flow in the veins in the initial phase
- venous flow then falls and disappears with full rigidity
- there is an increase in RI to >0.90 to indicate sufficient venous occlusion.

Indications for scanning

- Erectile dysfunction to detect impaired arterial inflow or venous leakage.
- High-resolution ultrasound to detect penile plaques in Peyronie's disease.
- Duplex flow characteristics as the preliminary investigation to diagnose the cause of priapism.

Criteria for diagnosing erectile dysfunction

Arteriogenic erectile dysfunction

In the flaccid penis, PSV <25–30 cm/s and AT >80 ms may be sufficient to make the diagnosis. During erection, arterial insufficiency is recognized by lack of dilatation and the normal increase of PSV in the proximal deep arteries of the penis, and an abnormal result is defined as PSV <30 cm/s.

Venous leakage

This is considered if arteries dilate and demonstrate adequately increased PSV but with an EDV >5 cm/s and reduction in the RI to <0.85.

PROTOCOLS FOR SCANNING

Prepare the patient

The investigation is very sensitive and usually best performed by a male sonographer. A serious attitude must be maintained. A doctor will be present if provocative tests are performed to produce an erection.

Select the best transducer

The penis is examined with a high-frequency linear array transducer. Power Doppler is particularly useful to show the anatomy of these small vessels. Perform a routine abdominal scan with a low-frequency curved or phased array transducer to examine the iliac arteries with particular emphasis on detecting IIA stenosis (see page 167 in Chapter 8).

Position the patient

Lay the patient supine with the penis placed dorsally on the pubic region. Rolled towels on either side may help to stabilize the penis.

Scanning techniques

Use colour Doppler to identify flow in all vessels and place the sample volume for spectral analysis to record flow velocities and other calculations.

Machine settings require a low wall filter, low colour PRF, and a colour map that displays slow flow.

Record the PSV and EDV in the aorta and each CIA and IIA. If present, calculate the severity of stenosis or extent of occlusion (see page 167 in Chapter 8).

Begin at the base of the flaccid penis.

- Obtain images in both transverse and longitudinal.
- Observe the echogenicity of the corpora cavernosa. They should be homogeneous throughout and increased echogenicity may indicate fibrosis due to Peyronie's disease.
- Measure the diameter of each cavernosal artery.
- Record a spectral signal and note the PSV and EDV in the cavernosal arteries. Calculate AT and RI.

If a vasoactive substance is given, the doctor will assess the clinical response. The patient is then rescanned as above. If tests are performed after stimulating an erection, then record the time intervals for noting results.

OTHER INVESTIGATIONS

Pulse volume recordings and penile/brachial pressure indices

Either photoplethysmography or CW Doppler can be used to measure the penile pressure distal to a narrow cuff at the base of the penis. A normal penile/brachial pressure index is >0.8 and an index <0.6 strongly suggests arteriogenic impotence.

Neurological investigations

Measurement of pudendal-evoked potentials and bulbocavernosal reflex times are used to distinguish patients with neurogenic impotence.

Arteriography

Selective internal iliac catheterization may be required to obtain penile arteriography to investigate causes of priapism.

Box 15.3: Ultrasound images to record

- Sample spectral traces of the aorta, CIAs and IIAs and at any stenosis.
- B-mode of the corpora cavernosa.
- B-mode diameters of cavernosal arteries pre- and post-stimulation.
- Sample spectral trace, AT and RI calculations in cavernosal arteries pre- and post-stimulation.
- Colour Doppler to show arterial and venous flow pre- and post-stimulation.

16

ULTRASOUND–GUIDED INTERVENTIONS

Various ultrasound techniques are available to guide interventions for arterial and venous disease. The following is not an exhaustive list.

MONITORING DURING ARTERIAL SURGERY

Some vascular surgeons use duplex scanning before final closure immediately after completing carotid endarterectomy or infrainguinal vein bypass to detect technical problems causing haemodynamic abnormalities such as flaps, kinks, a twisted graft, retained valves after *in situ* bypass, or residual stenosis. Reintervention occurs in at least 5 per cent of operations.

For **carotid endarterectomy**, severe abnormalities in the ICA and CCA include raised PSV – ICA PSV > 50 cm/s or ICA/CCA PSV ratio >3.0, or B-mode evidence of a flap ⩾2 mm long, dissection, narrowing, kinking, or thrombus. Any of these warrant immediate revision, This reduces the risk of perioperative stroke and late restenosis. Duplex scanning is more accurate than intra-operative angiography.

For an **infrainguinal bypass**, PSV > 80 cm/s, spectral broadening, velocity ratio > 3.0, kinking, twist or thrombus indicate the need for revision to improve early patency rates. A PSV < 30–40 cm/s and absent diastolic flow suggest the need for a distal arteriovenous fistula or sequential distal bypass graft to augment flow. Any abnormality may be an indication for aggressive post-operative antithrombotic treatment.

ENDOVASCULAR TREATMENT OF OCCLUSIVE ARTERIAL DISEASE

It is traditional to perform balloon dilatation or stenting under fluoroscopic control in a radiology suite. However, these procedures can be performed with a combination of B-mode to show passage of the guidewires, catheters and balloons, and colour and spectral Doppler to identify stenosis or occlusion and confirm that it has been restored towards normal by treatment. This is best suited to the accessible femoropopliteal arterial segment.

TREATMENT OF PSEUDOANEURYSMS

Pseudoaneurysms now most often result from arterial puncture and insertion of a sheath in the common femoral artery during coronary angiography or cardiac endovascular treatment (Fig. 16.1). Conservative ultrasound-guided techniques can permanently occlude the aneurysm so as to avoid open surgical repair.

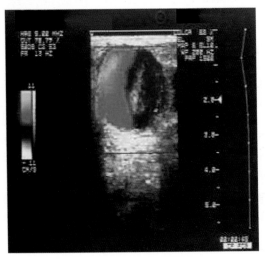

Fig. 16.1
Colour Doppler image of a pseudoaneurysm
Swirling flow in the aneurysm produces the 'ying-yang sign'.

Ultrasound-guided compression

Pressure is applied at a strategic point to occlude the connection from the artery to the aneurysm so that stasis within the aneurysm causes it to thrombose. This is effective in over 75 per cent, but the process frequently needs to be repeated, and each session can take up to 60 min so that it is very taxing to the patient and sonographer. Success is less likely if the neck is wide, the aneurysm is large or long-standing, if there is considerable pain making it difficult to maintain compression, or if the patient is anticoagulated.

Ultrasound-guided thrombin injection

This is an attractive alternative to compression. Under local anaesthesia, a 20-gauge needle is placed in the aneurysm well away from the neck, and human thrombin is injected slowly until the aneurysm occludes. Colour Doppler and B-mode scanning show the process well. The aneurysm is almost always permanently controlled within a few minutes at the first treatment, even in anticoagulated patients. However, local arterial or venous thrombosis and pulmonary embolism have been reported as occasional complications.

THROMBOLYTIC THERAPY

Thrombolysis, for example to treat a thrombosed haemodialysis access graft, can be monitored outside the fluoroscopy suite using B-mode and colour Doppler to confirm that flow is re-established. It is frequently necessary after successful lysis to treat underlying stenosis by balloon dilatation, stenting, or surgery.

TREATMENT OF CHRONIC VENOUS DISEASE

Ultrasound-guided sclerotherapy

Traditional treatment for varicose veins by surgical ligation and stripping has been supplemented in recent years by ultrasound-guided sclerotherapy (UGS) of the saphenous trunk. Planning

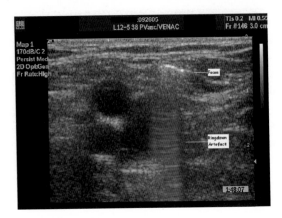

Fig. 16.2

B-mode showing foam in the saphenous vein and superficial tributaries after ultrasound-guided sclerotherapy

Note the ringdown artefact deep to the foam.

treatment requires a careful pre-operative venous duplex study (see Chapter 10).

The outcome has been improved by techniques to prepare foamed sclerosants. Foam largely displaces blood from the lumen and immediately causes the vein to spasm so that less thrombus develops. Foam is highly echogenic for ultrasound, allowing precise placement of an appropriate volume to fill the full length of the affected saphenous vein and its tributaries (Fig. 16.2). Foam does not flow as a liquid sclerosant would so that it stays in contact with the vein wall for up to 30 min after injection and this allows sclerosant to be diluted since it will be acting for much longer than liquid sclerosant.

Injection techniques

A tilt table is used with reverse Trendelenburg to 30°. This makes it more simple to puncture the vein and also keeps foam distally within superficial veins until injection is completed. Foam causes such intense spasm that the vein does not fill with blood in treated segments despite being dependent. When superficial veins have been filled, the sonographer flattens the table and compresses the

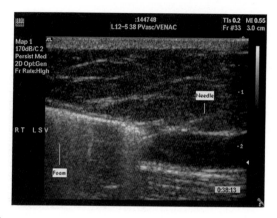

Fig. 16.3

B-mode showing foam being injected into the great saphenous vein during ultrasound-guided sclerotherapy

saphenous junction for 2–3 min to prevent excess foam passing to the deep veins.

There are several approaches for UGS.

Saphenous puncture

Inject as far distal to the saphenous junction as possible where the diameter is still sufficient for the vein to be easily punctured. Hold the transducer exactly perpendicular to the skin to show the vein in longitudinal to guide the needle, and place the needle exactly in the midline of the transducer axis to show its full length and foam in the vein as it is injected (Fig. 16.3). An alternative approach is to hold the transducer to show the vein in transverse and approach with the needle from one or other side. This allows the transducer to be shifted up or down to bring the needle into view if it has not been placed correctly, but it does not show any length of the vein. Foam is injected slowly and the screen is watched to confirm it is flowing along the vein, and injection is immediately stopped if extravasation is seen.

Injection through tributaries

This is used if the limb has large tributaries. The sonographer follows foam to confirm it is passing in the desired direction, and if not then compresses the vein to direct flow into other varicosities. Large thigh and calf perforators are compressed by the transducer or by a finger.

Injection into tributaries with ultrasound guidance may be necessary for a superficial tributary that is not clearly visible. The most common reason is to obliterate tributaries draining from incompetent perforators. A site is chosen to inject the tributary as far distal to a perforator as possible to attempt to prevent foamed sclerosant entering a deep vein through the perforator. The transducer is then shifted to the perforator site, injection is stopped as soon as foam is seen at its superficial end, and digital compression is applied for 2–3 min. The procedure may need to be repeated for a tributary proximal to the perforator.

Ultrasound-guided endovenous laser therapy or radiofrequency closure

These are favoured by some phlebologists for larger diameter saphenous veins. The vein is punctured as far distally as possible, and either a laser probe or radiofrequency probe are passed along the vein to just below the saphenous junction (Fig. 16.4). The position

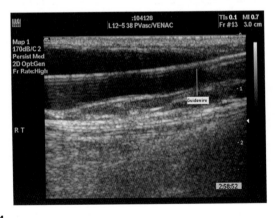

Fig. 16.4

B-mode showing a guidewire inserted into the great saphenous vein during ultrasound-guided endovenous laser therapy

of the probe tip is confirmed by B-mode. The entire length from the saphenous junction to the puncture site is destroyed as the activated probe is withdrawn.

Ultrasound-guided sclerotherapy for venous malformations

Surgery to treat a vascular malformation commonly causes extensive damage, major bleeding and incomplete excision. Sclerotherapy is an alternative treatment, now usually using foamed sclerosant which is clearly seen with B-mode.

NEEDLE AND CATHETER PLACEMENT

Conventional ultrasound can be used to guide a femoral puncture for arteriography or endovascular intervention, to shorten the time taken and increase success rates, particularly for difficult cases with common femoral disease or obesity. Needles with an ultrasound crystal at the tip have been used.

Various intravenous catheters can be inserted under ultrasound control, usually through veins from the upper limbs for intravenous drug or nutritional therapy, administration of blood products, withdrawal of blood, or physiological monitoring. Ultrasound can be used to detect complications, particularly infection or thrombosis.

Central venous catheters

Central venous catheters are favoured for long-term use, such as for parenteral nutrition, but their insertion can cause damage to major vessels in the neck and mediastinum. A central venous line is inserted through the subclavian, internal jugular, axillary or femoral veins with the tip in the superior vena cava or right atrium. Catheters can be placed percutaneously and not tunnelled, partially implanted and tunnelled, or implanted totally subcutaneously. The subclavian vein has been the insertion site of choice and this usually requires operating theatre facilities. However, ultrasound guidance is effective for percutaneous puncture of the internal jugular or axillary vein, particularly in complicated cases, for example with obesity or dyspnoea. For axillary puncture, ultrasound is used to examine the vein from below the mid-clavicular point.

Peripheral venous catheters

The peripheral route can be used for infusions for shorter periods and these reduce risks.

- **Peripherally inserted central catheters (PICC lines)** are inserted through the cephalic, basilic or brachial veins.
- **Peripheral access system (PAS) ports** are inserted through forearm veins.

These avoid the risk of major vascular trauma during insertion and can be placed outside an operating theatre. However, they are more prone to cause mechanical phlebitis, venous thrombosis, infection or catheter fracture if left in for more than a few days, and these complications are well detected by ultrasound (Fig. 16.5). The optimal tip location is in the superior vena cava and this is best confirmed with an anteroposterior chest X-ray.

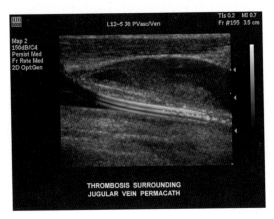

Fig. 16.5

B-mode showing thrombus around an intravenous catheter

INTRAVASCULAR ULTRASOUND (IVUS)

The technology is rapidly improving, currently with fine 3.5 F catheters and high-frequency 20 MHz transducers available for B-mode and colour Doppler imaging. IVUS is being increasingly used for peripheral arterial or venous and coronary arterial interventions to show the vessel lumen and wall, branches and tributaries and surrounding structures. This avoids radiation and contrast toxicity resulting from conventional fluoroscopic control. IVUS requires additional equipment and personnel, and the expense of disposable probes but it can be cost-effective. It has been used in several situations for peripheral vascular disease.

Intervention for stenotic or occlusive arterial disease

Intra-operative IVUS helps to:

- demonstrate complex anatomy and unclear findings from arteriography
- determine whether plaque is non-calcified or calcified, and eccentric or concentric
- accurately measure arterial diameters and the extent of disease to select proper angioplasty balloon size
- confirm full expansion and attachment to the arterial wall for a stent or stent graft
- detect arterial rupture, intimal flaps and dissection after balloon dilatation
- show residual flaps or thrombus after endarterectomy.

Post-operative IVUS has been used to assess late recurrence due to further atherosclerosis or neointimal hyperplasia.

Endovascular aneurysm repair (EVAR)

Intra-operative IVUS accurately measures aortic diameters to select the best sized stent-graft and this helps to reduce the frequency of type I endoleaks (see Chapter 8). It alters the selection of graft size in approximately one-third of patients where size was calculated from a pre-operative CT scan. IVUS can assess outcome without completion arteriography to ensure that renal or suprarenal artery orifices have not been covered, and to detect potential endoleaks.

Endovascular treatment of aortic dissection

EVAR and fenestration of the dissection flap improve vessel perfusion to relieve visceral or lower limb ischaemia, and occlude the intimal entry tear, decrease pressure and initiate thrombosis within the false lumen to reduce the risk of aneurysmal dilatation. IVUS has been used with other imaging modalities to stage dissections after initial stabilization. IVUS helps to guide placement of a stent-graft and select the site for fenestration.

Diagnosis and endovascular treatment for vena cava or iliac vein compression

IVUS is used to diagnose the cause of extrinsic major venous compression or intrinsic venous stenosis and associated thrombosis, and to direct guidewire placement and endovascular treatment by balloon dilatation or stenting.

Inferior vena cava filter placement

IVUS can be used to guide insertion of an inferior vena cava filter in the intensive care unit. A single groin puncture is used for both IVUS and filter placement. Major branch veins, thrombosis, and caval diameter and the ideal site for filter location are demonstrated without the need for contrast agents.

RECOMMENDED READING

Gent R. 1997: *Applied Physics and Technology of Diagnostic Ultrasound.* Available from: Department of Paediatric Ultrasound, Women's and Children's Hospital, Adelaide, South Australia, Australia, 5006.

Hobson RW, Wilson SE, Veith FJ. 2003: *Vascular Surgery: Principles and Practice,* 3rd edn. New York: Marcel Dekker.

Strandness DE. 2001: *Duplex Scanning in Vascular Disorders,* 2nd edn. Philadelphia: Lippincott, Williams and Wilkins.

Zwiebel WJ. 2004: *Introduction to Vascular Ultrasonography,* 5th edn. Philadelphia: WB Saunders.

INDEX

Page numbers in **bold** type refer to figures; those in *italics* to tables and boxed material